SELF-ASSESSMEN
STUDENT NURSES

SELF-ASSESSMENT FOR STUDENT NURSES

Edited by
JOYCE ARTHURS B.Ed(Hons) RGN SCM Dip.N RNT Cert.Ed.
Nurse Tutor
The General Infirmary
Leeds

PASTEST SERVICE
Hemel Hempstead
Hertfordshire England

© 1986 PASTEST SERVICE
304 Galley Hill
Hemel Hempstead, Hertfordshire HP1 3LE

British Library Cataloguing in Publication Data
Arthurs, Joyce
   Self assessment for student nurses: patient profiles, and objective test questions, answers, explanations and marking system.
   1. Nursing — Problems, exercises, etc.
   I. Title
   610.73'076   RT55

   ISBN 0-906896-50-9

Text prepared on a microcomputer by Turner Associates, Knutsford.
Phototypeset by Communitype, Leicester.
Printed by Oxford University Press.

CONTENTS

Brackets indicate the number of patient profiles in each category. Each profile has 3 or 4 related questions.

A LETTER FROM THE EDITOR

Dear Reader

This book has been produced to assist student and pupil nurses who are preparing for their final examinations. It is also of relevance to all those returning to nursing after several years of absence whether raising a family or for whatever reason.

Over the last few years there has been a considerable change in emphasis in nurse education from task orientation to total patient care and the questions chosen here reflect this change. We live in a changing world, and the State Final Examination in its present form will soon be a thing of the past, however the usefulness of a self-assessment book like this one remains undiminished.

The patient profiles and objective test questions chosen for this book were carefully selected from over 600 submitted by experienced nurse tutors all over the country and these questions were then extensively edited, pre-tested and validated before finally being included.

The notes at the beginning have been written on the basis of many years experience helping nurse learners to prepare for their professional examinations and I would like to stress that some time spent reading over these introductory pages will prove well worthwhile.

I would also like to convey a word of thanks to the many people who have assisted in the preparation of this book, especially the tutors who wrote initial questions and answers for editing, and the student and pupil nurses and teachers who were so helpful with the pre-testing. I am most grateful to you all.

Finally may I wish you every success in your chosen career of nursing, both as a learner and when you become registered or enrolled.

Joyce Arthurs
Nurse Tutor
The General Infirmary
Leeds.

HOW TO USE THIS BOOK

The questions presented here were written with The Nursing Process and a problem-solving approach in mind. We have included questions on many different aspects of care relating to patients of different ages with a variety of problems, both acute and chronic. Each question has been pre-tested by being answered by approximately 100 nurses. The initials (EN) after the patient profile denote questions tested by senior pupil nurses, and (RGN) indicates that senior student nurses tested the question. Of the 58 patient profiles in this book 19 are marked (EN) and 39 (RGN) and they are accompanied by 213 related objective test questions.

This book has been set out broadly following Roper's Activities of Living. A short profile is given of a patient in a particular situation, followed by three or four questions relating to that patient. Do not forget that like most multiple choice questions for nurses there is only *one* correct answer to each question.

Questions are printed on the right-hand page, with the correct answers and explanations on the following page. Alongside each answer you will find a percentage figure which indicates the number of finalist nurses who chose the correct answer during pre-testing the questions. Questions with a high percentage are easier than those with a low percentage. By using this information you will be able to identify areas which need concentrated revision. It will also enable you to assess your own level of performance relative to that of other finalists.

In order for you to be able to test your own level of knowledge there is a line at the bottom of each question page in which you should write your own answers before turning over. In this way you can then work through each section of the book coming back to mark your own answers as right or wrong by checking against the correct answers and explanations given on the following page.

The teaching explanations provided are very important as an aid to study. If you get the question right you should have got it right for the right reasons and not just a guess. If you answered it wrongly then the explanations should help you to decide why you made the error. Do not forget that the questions are of varying degrees of difficulty. For example, if only 40% of learners were successful at pre-testing a particular question, do not be too disheartened if your answer is not correct. If, however, the figure given is 95% you should find this question easy if you have studied this area. Finally as a revision aid you can go through the book later picking out all the questions that you got wrong (easily visible by your markings at the bottom of each page) and you can use this method to identify areas which still need further study.

Be sure to mark your answers clearly in the spaces provided at the bottom of each page, for example:

Mark your answers here: 94...C...95...B...96...A...97...B...
                              ✓   ✓   ✗   ✓

and in this way you can later correct your answers and look at the explanations given overleaf.

This book can be used to *dip into* throughout your training. For example, after a period of medical nursing, a learner at the end of his/her first year should be able to answer some of the questions relating to problems encountered by patients on a medical ward. Thus, by the end of your basic education, you should be able to answer correctly most of the questions in the book. EN questions for pupil nurses, EN and RGN questions for student nurses.

Alternatively leave the questions until the end of training, by which time student nurses and many pupils should be able to go straight through the pages successfully answering most of the questions.

THE COMPETENCIES REQUIRED
FOR REGISTRATION

Nurse training leading to qualification as a first level nurse shall provide opportunities to enable the student to accept responsibility for her personal professional development and to acquire the competencies required to

a)   advise on the promotion of health and the prevention of illness;

b)   recognise situations that may be detrimental to the health and wellbeing of the individual;

c)   carry out those activities involved when conducting the comprehensive assessment of a person's nursing requirements;

d)   recognise the significance of the observations made and use these to develop an initial nursing assessment;

e)   devise a plan of nursing care based on the assessment with the co-operation of the patient, to the extent that this is possible, taking into account the medical prescription;

f)   implement the planned programme of nursing care and where appropriate teach and co-ordinate other members of the caring team who may be responsible for implementing specific aspects of the nursing care;

g)   review the effectiveness of the nursing care provided, and where appropriate, initiate any action that may be required;

h)   work in a team with other nurses, and with medical and para-medical staff and social workers;

i)   undertake the management of the care of a group of patients over a period of time and organise the appropriate support services; related to the care of the particular type of patient with whom she is likely to come in contact when registered in that part of the register for which the student intends to qualify.

* The preceding list of competencies are reproduced from The Nurses, Midwives and Health Visitors Rules Approval Order, Stat. Instrument No. 873 by permission of the United Kingdom Central Council.

THE TECHNIQUE OF STUDYING EFFECTIVELY

In order to use study time as effectively as possible, the choosing of a suitable environment is vital. Each individual must also consider his or her own physical needs as these work hand in hand with environmental requirements.

Here are some general guidelines which may be helpful. The room must be adequately illuminated, by available light during the day and by suitable shadow-free light during the hours of darkness. Many people find it helpful to use a straight-backed chair when working at a desk or table, especially if they are making notes or writing essays. A comfortable arm-chair after a large meal is unlikely to be very stimulating. Wherever possible books should be left on the table between study sessions, although this may only be possible if a special study room is available or if the family are prepared to tolerate this inconvenience. The temperature of the room is important; the student in her overcoat crouched over an open fire in a freezing cold room will not be able to work efficiently and the overheated stuffy atmosphere in some nurses' homes is equally unsuitable! Many people find that a cool room with adequate ventilation is best for study.

The acceptable level of noise in a room depends on the individual. Some people need total quiet whilst others find that background music aids concentration. However, loud irregular noises are almost always distracting, and if the next-door neighbour is a DIY enthusiast using a drill or hammer then studying becomes very hard indeed. If one has difficulty finding somewhere suitable to study, the local public library or the School of Nursing library may be a good place to take refuge. In summer it may be possible to study in the open air, in the garden or some part of the hospital grounds, but for some this can prove distracting.

Many people experience problems in concentrating if they are not physically alert. How often do students have difficulty keeping awake in lectures after lunch? Studying when hungry, thirsty, tired, uncomfortable or under the weather is often not very productive, and these factors should be considered if the best use is to be made of the time available. Owls find it better to study at night, but larks are at their best in the morning; so each person should discover his/her optimum time of day to study. Adequate rest and recreation are essential during a course of study, and students who omit rest days and do not treat themselves occasionally often find their work becomes less productive in terms of learning.

It is important to appreciate that the attention span is often shorter than people realise. A short break every 20 to 30 minutes is helpful, even if it means simply glancing up from the work, stretching and looking out of the window for a few minutes. Making a drink is also a good way of resting the mind for a short time at a suitable point during the session.

As well as considering the environmental and physical factors required by an individual, the learner must also take into account other features that determine a *planned* approach to study. To illustrate this point one must listen to the complaints of nurse tutors many of whom say that learners do not use information from one area when studying another. For instance; if an 83 year old lady, recently widowed, comes into hospital for a routine operation, then nurses plan care for this lady based on the problems caused by her condition. However, when she is being assessed the nurses may not use their knowledge about the special needs of the elderly and the bereaved when writing their care plan. It is difficult but important for nurses to use their previously acquired knowledge when studying a new topic, and they must avoid developing compartments in the mind which, like sealed boxes, can only be opened when the appropriate signal is given.

Learning is much easier if the new skill or information is used. Unless one is a collector of useless information, facts and skills which are not used may soon become forgotten because they are seen as irrelevant and useless. For this reason, nurses should plan their private study in conjunction with the programme in the School of Nursing, and the practical work on the wards. In this way, not only does their work become more effective, it also becomes relevant to real life and much more interesting.

PLANNING YOUR COURSE OF STUDY

A good way to work and learn effectively is to make a detailed study plan for personal use and to keep to it throughout the training period. By forming good study habits, assessments and examinations can be approached with confidence. The plan does not have to be rigidly adhered to but the student should be honest with herself, and missed study sessions really should be made up by an extra effort later.

At the beginning of their training learners may be given an overall plan, and this, along with information about care studies, timing of assessments, holidays etc, forms the basis of the study plan. If this information is not provided, it should be freely available from the course tutor and should be obtained as soon as possible.

The next step is to decide on how many hours each week can realistically be devoted to study. At this stage many people grossly overestimate and are very disappointed when they cannot meet their targets. Thus it is often better to aim low and to exceed the time expected. A suggested starting point is about five hours each week, possibly falling to three hours some weeks, and compensating by having *heavy* weeks of seven hours or more. The actual topic for study can be selected in relation to the overall plan of training. For example, a typical training module might start with a study week about care of the elderly, followed by ten weeks on the geriatric ward before a second week in school. During the clinical experience the nurse may have a care study to complete before the second study block. It would be a good plan to spend the first 3-4 weeks expanding knowledge gained in school, and the rest of the time writing the care study and doing some preparatory reading for the next study block. This would also mean that the topic is being related directly to the clinical experience. However, do not forget to build rest days and short breaks from studying into your overall plan.

SOME LEARNING RESOURCES

In the School of Nursing

The School of Nursing Syllabus and the list of competencies drawn up by the UKCC for nurses to achieve before registration (quoted in full on page 5), are useful resources. These can be used as the framework for private study throughout the nurse's training (along the lines suggested in the previous chapter) and also act as a *check list* to ensure that nothing has been omitted from the study plan.

The major resource available to help the student in the School of Nursing is the Tutor. Tutors often spend time with individual students offering help and guidance with all aspects of the student's world. They can suggest other resources to help with study, and can monitor an individual's progress by marking extra work and discussing specific problems. These problems may be related to work or may be of a personal nature and the Tutor can often offer practical help in difficult situations.

One specific way in which Tutors can help is to use, for example, learning games as learning experiences which help people identify their strengths and weaknesses. In this way students can congratulate themselves when good marks are achieved, and can also identify weak subject areas where further study is needed.

Tutors often provide handouts or lecture notes, which are of great value when reviewing material at a later date. The old joke, A lecture is a session where information passes from the notes of the lecturer to the notes of the students, without passing through the brains of either, is only true if the students (and teachers) are content to allow this to happen. Re-reading, and writing up lecture notes are often very efficient ways to learn.

Many other activities centred on the school are valuable learning experiences which can be followed up during private study. Discussions and group tutorials can stimulate further reading and development of informed opinions. Projects such as care studies can lead to exploration in many areas, and usually, the more effort the student puts in to these, the greater the rewards in terms of learning.

On the Ward

Nurse learners often say that they learn most on the ward, when actually nursing patients. It is common for nurses to remember 'Mrs so-and-so' with her particular problems, and how these were overcome; these experiences then become reference points for nursing other patients with

9

similar problems. This kind of learning, however, has one great disadvantage: students often assume that the way things are done at their hospital is the only way. This is a dangerous misconception which arises from the person's own inexperience, but a good way to avoid it is to supplement clinical practice with reading and private study. Of course it is a good idea to study the way that patients are nursed at the training hospital, and to learn from that experience, and there are several agencies which can help. The nursing and medical records of patients will reveal the story of their illnesses, and should include an account of care given and an evaluation of that care. Nurses working on the ward, and the clinical teacher who liaises with the school, can all help by adding their wide experience to the learner's knowledge, and part of their job is to help teach students. Most nurses are only too pleased to help, but because of the pressure of work it may be left to the student to approach them at a quiet time on the ward. Nurses who show interest by asking relevant questions usually find that others are very willing to help.

In the Library

The School of Nursing Library is a learning resource, but it is sometimes sadly underused. In order to use the library efficiently, the student must be familiar with the index system used and library staff are generally willing to explain this.

When studying a particular topic it is important to refer to a number of different sources, and the library will have a wide range of useful material if only the student knows how to locate it! Library staff are usually very happy to help once they are aware of the learner's interest and particular need.

The library will also contain many of the nursing journals, and students should put aside some time, each week if possible, to scan these magazines for useful material for study and also to keep up to date with new trends and nursing politics.

All students will need to buy a small number of textbooks; a nursing dictionary, physiology book, and a good nursing text are essential. If the school does not require the student to buy *set* books, then the library is a good place to view a selection before buying the one most suited to the individual's preference. It will save money if books which will only be used for a limited period are borrowed from the library, rather than bought. One last word, only use *recent* publications, and beware of buying secondhand books.

Other resources

There are many other sources which can provide nursing students with useful information. Groups which exist to help people with particular problems, e.g. The Mastectomy Association, 'Headway', and Age Concern, are examples of associations whose representatives can often give outsiders insight into the particular difficulties of members. Local Health Education Centres, Town Hall Health Departments and DHSS offices are also places where additional help and pamphlets may be found by the enquiring student.

USING THE NURSING PROCESS
AND NURSING MODELS

The Nursing Process is perhaps best described as a way of organising the care given to patients, which can be broken down into four stages: assessing, planning, implementing and evaluating.

Using The Nursing Process has helped change the emphasis in the delivery of care from a series of specific tasks (such as pressure area care, or looking after all the intravenous infusions) to the care of the *whole* patient.

A further development has been that of Nursing Models, and these provide the framework for the use of The Nursing Process. Nursing Models are many and varied, but a popular model was developed in the United Kingdom by Roper, Logan and Tierney. This focuses on different functions which healthy people perform in everyday life, such as breathing, mobilising, and sleeping. The assessment stage of The Nursing Process involves identifying problems which the patient experiences, or may experience, in these areas. The nurse then plans her work to help alleviate or prevent these problems and then, when the planned care has been given, she evaluates its success before re-planning her subsequent attention to that patient. For example, many patients have problems mobilising, which may mean that they are at risk of developing pressure sores (potential problem assessed). The nurse plans to help the patient change position two hourly, and this is done for 24 hours (planning and implementing care), before observing the patient for early signs that a sore may develop (evaluating). This highly simplified example has been used to show the reader how the practice of The Nursing Process (with whichever Model is used in the training hospital), should be carried over into theoretical work and studying.

A very good way to organise your study is to work through the steps of The Nursing Process with a typical (imaginary) patient suffering from a disease at a certain stage. Of course, if a real patient is available to study, then so much the better. In situations such as the above, the nurse must take into account factors such as the age and sex of the patient, together with the social circumstances and their level of education and understanding.

Example 1

Brian Wolfenden, aged three years is about to be discharged from hospital following a severe head injury which he sustained when he was knocked over by a car. His parents are both school teachers and they say that Brian has fully recovered except that he cannot speak as well as he could before his accident. Brian's grandmother usually looks after him while his parents are at work.

Example 2

Miss Wendy Ripley, a 75 year old lady, is admitted to your ward for geriatric assessment. She had a left-sided stroke 6 months ago and is having difficulty managing at home, even with a home help and 'Meals-on-Wheels'. Miss Ripley has no relatives but refuses to give up her home.

Could you assess the care needed by these people? How would you do this? Could you write a plan for nursing them and devise a strategy for evaluating the care you would give?

Why not have a try, using a Nursing Model with which you are familiar.

1 : EATING AND DRINKING

Mary Jones is 12 years old and has been admitted to hospital for stabilisation of her recently diagnosed diabetes mellitus because out-patient treatment was not achieving this. Her father is a long distance lorry driver and her mother works part-time as a morning cashier. Mary has two younger sisters.(EN)

1   Which of the following would most likely have caused Mary's mother to seek medical advice for her daughter. Mary had

   A   polyuria and polydipsia
   B   polydipsia and enuresis
   C   polyuria and weight gain
   D   polydipsia and weight gain

2   Mary is prescribed insulin for her condition. Which of the following is the most appropriate when teaching Mary and her parents about Mary's care. To

   A   teach Mary and her parents at separate times
   B   limit the teaching session to half an hour
   C   explain the disease in great detail
   D   provide adequate time for questions

3   Mary will be subjected to a hypoglycaemic state in a controlled environment in order to ensure that

   A   her parents are aware of the signs that Mary exhibits
   B   Mary knows what hypoglycaemia feels like
   C   her parents always provide an adequate diet
   D   Mary does not give herself too much insulin

4   The most appropriate advice regarding Mary's clothes is that her parents should

   A   ensure she wears a sweater at all times to prevent chilling
   B   check her shoes frequently to see they fit properly
   C   ensure that Mary avoids woollen clothes to prevent skin irritation
   D   ensure she wears lightweight clothes to prevent sweating

Mark your answers here: 1.......2.......3.......4.......

15

1 **A   67%**

The most common first sign of diabetes mellitus is the increased urinary output (polyuria) due to the excess glucose excreted in the urine. To maintain the body's fluid balance the person will be thirsty and increase the fluid intake (polydipsia).

2 **D   82%**

One of the basic principles of teaching is to permit two way flow of information and feedback. Therefore time must be allowed for expansion and clarification of information. Teaching of care to a child of Mary's age is best done together, so that both parent and child can learn and appreciate what is involved. Some sessions may take longer than half an hour if there are many questions or if everyone is trying out the procedure. The amount of detail which is required and is appropriate will vary.

3 **B   81%**

It is *most* important that Mary is aware of how she feels if she has a hypoglycaemic attack. She will then be able to take the appropriate action, or indicate that others should do so.

4 **B   75%**

This aspect of care is *most* important in the care of a person who has diabetes. Peripheral neuritis and vascular complications are the main complications. Her shoes must be fitted properly and changed as soon as they become even slightly too small. Foot hygiene should also be emphasised. C: unless Mary is allergic to wool this will not happen. In fact, man-made fibre is less absorbent and more likely to cause a rash due to a build-up of sweat. D is not a practical suggestion. At certain times of the year thick clothes are appropriate, and in hot weather sweating is a normal way to maintain the body's natural temperature, so the basic concept inferred in this statement is incorrect.

55KGS = 8St

Mr George Peters, a 48 year old builder with a history of an acquired inguinal hernia, has been admitted to your ward for emergency surgery because of strangulation of the hernia. He smokes 60 cigarettes a day and weighs 93 kilograms. Mr Peters has experienced pain for the last week and yesterday afternoon whilst lifting a girder he had sudden severe pain and by evening he was vomiting. On admission at 07.00 hours he has vomiting, diarrhoea and pain.(EN)

5   Which of the following would give most reassurance to Mrs Peters who is very anxious about her husband's condition:

A   tell her that surgery will soon put the matter right
B   explain in lay terms exactly what a strangulated hernia is
C   make an appointment for Mrs Peters to see the surgeon later
D   give Mrs Peters the ward telephone number and advise her when to ring

6   Which of the following would be most effective in reducing Mr Peters' vomiting:

A   administer the prescribed antiemetic four hourly
B   give a mouth wash to reduce the nausea
C   ask Mr Peters to take deep breaths through his mouth
D   pass a nasogastric tube and aspirate the stomach contents hourly

7   Which of the following pieces of advice is most likely to prevent recurrence of Mr Peters' hernia in the future:

A   reduce weight by taking less carbohydrate
B   when coughing support the suture line
C   gradually increase abdominal exercise and avoid strain
D   do not return to work for three months

Mark your answers here: 5.......6.......7.......

5   B   66%

Each of the four actions is necessary, however, reassurance can only be given if we give certainty by stating exactly what has happened and how the condition occurred.

6   D   50%

Only by removing the accumulating fluid from the stomach can vomiting be reduced.

7   C   66%

It is essential to improve muscle tone gradually but also to avoid strain in the future. As this is a congenital weakness it is very likely to recur. The other options (A,B,D) are important to the plan of care but ineffective without C.

Mrs Rita Smith, aged 55 years, is a widow and school teacher. Her past history includes pernicious anaemia for which she is being treated. She is not interested in her food and has lost 2 stones during the last 3 months. She says that even when she is hungry after a very small meal she feels she has eaten too much. She is diagnosed as suffering from carcinoma of the stomach.(EN)

8   During her first 24 hours in hospital whilst you are with her she has a severe haematemesis. Which of the following actions would be most helpful to Mrs Smith:

   A   lie her down and elevate the foot of the bed
   B   stay with her and give her support and comfort
   C   go and call the nurse in charge
   D   prepare the equipment for a transfusion

9   Which of the following drugs will Mrs Smith be given for her pernicious anaemia:

   A   cyanocobalamine
   B   ferrous gluconate
   C   ferrous sulphate
   D   carbimazole

10   Which of the following would you expect on the third post-total-gastrectomy day when you are aspirating Mrs Smith's nasogastric tube:

   A   approximately 50 ml of acidic fluid
   B   about 300 ml in 24 hours
   C   very little or no aspirate
   D   a small amount of acid fluid

11   While you are bathing Mrs Smith she says "I have got a cancer haven't I?" Which of the following would be the most suitable reply:

   A   "I'm not sure I'll ask the doctor for you"
   B   "Would you like to talk to the sister about it?"
   C   "Yes you have, do you want to see the chaplain?"
   D   "What is it that makes you say that?"

Mark your answers here: 8.......9........10.......11.......

8 **B** **58%**

The most helpful action for Mrs Smith is to stay with her and give her support and comfort. You can use the call bell and obtain assistance at the same time.

9 **A** **61%**

Failure to absorb vitamin B_{12} is the cause of pernicious anaemia therefore only cyanocobalamine can be used to treat it.

10 **C** **65%**

There would be little or no aspirate as there is no longer a reservoir for fluid or food and peristalsis should have re-commenced.

11 **D** **68%**

All except for C and D are evasive, C is cruel since she may be hoping she has been wrong in her assumption and does not wish for spiritual help. D helps to discover what she really knows so that she can be helped from that point.

Mrs Mary Staut, a middle-aged mother of two teenage children is admitted to the medical ward suffering from severe pernicious anaemia. She is to have a transfusion of concentrated red cells.(EN)

12 Which of the following groups of features will Mrs Staut have most likely suffered from:

   A   pallor, weight loss, cyanosis
   B   pallor, tiredness, cyanosis
   C   weight loss, breathlessness, cyanosis
   D   pallor, breathlessness, tiredness

13 Which of the following describes the reason for the deficiency of vitamin B_{12} in the body, which causes pernicious anaemia:

   A   deficiency of the vitamin in the normal dietary intake
   B   failure to absorb the vitamin due to a lack of intrinsic factor
   C   vitamin B_{12} is destroyed by an excess of hydrochloric acid
   D   failure to absorb the vitamin due to failure of fat absorption

14 Mrs Staut asks you whether the tingling that she has noticed in her hands and feet over the previous few weeks has anything to do with her anaemia. Which of the following would be the most appropriate reply:

   A   it may well be connected, and will not get any worse now she is having treatment
   B   it is not connected to the anaemia and should be investigated
   C   it is probably connected but she should report the fact to the doctor in case it needs investigation
   D   it is a nerve manifestation of the anaemia and will disappear now she is having treatment

15 Mrs Staut will need to continue with vitamin B_{12} therapy on a long-term basis. This treatment is provided by

   A   a daily intake of intrinsic factor
   B   monthly injections of vitamin B_{12}
   C   daily injections of vitamin B_{12}
   D   weekly injections of intrinsic factor

Mark your answers here: 12.......13.......14.......15.......

12   D   70%

As with all anaemias, the principal features are those described in D. Cyanosis is not a feature of anaemia as cyanosis is due to the presence of large amounts of deoxygenated haemoglobin. In anaemia, the problem is due to insufficient haemoglobin, so pallor is common but cyanosis rare. Weight loss is not common despite gastrointestinal disturbances.

13   B   90%

The intrinsic factor which is secreted by the stomach, in the presence of hydrochloric acid combines with vitamin B_{12} and provides for its absorption in the small intestine. Most patients with pernicious anaemia suffer from an absence of hydrochloric acid (achlorhydria).

14   C   75%

Over 80% of patients with pernicious anaemia have some sort of neurological sign or symptom before seeking treatment and this may well be the cause of Mrs Staut's 'tingling'. The medical staff may wish to investigate and the facts should be reported to them.

15   B   76%

As vitamin B_{12} cannot be absorbed by the digestive tract, it will need to be given by injection. Following an initial period of more frequent injections (e.g. weekly), the long-term therapy is usually *monthly* injections. Intrinsic factor cannot be given.

Mrs Joan Firth, a 55 year old widow, is admitted to your ward suffering from anaemia and paraesthesia of her toes. The doctors diagnose pernicious anaemia with early neurological involvement. Her haemoglobin is 6.5 g/100 ml on admission.(RGN)

16   The cause of pernicious anaemia is

    A   prolonged minor blood loss
    B   prolonged treatment with anticonvulsants
    C   vitamin B_{12} deficiency
    D   malabsorption of vitamin B_{12}

17   Which of the following should be included in Mrs Firth's care for the first few days in hospital:

    A   strict bed-rest with controlled visiting
    B   bed-rest with a commode for toilet purposes
    C   getting up for meals and toilet only
    D   allowing Mrs Firth to care for herself

18   The definitive test for pernicious anaemia is

    A   the Schilling test
    B   packed cell volume
    C   haemoglobin estimation
    D   bone marrow biopsy

19   Mrs Firth is worried about her long-term future. The most appropriate information to give her is that

    A   she will have to wait and see how much improvement results from the treatment
    B   pernicious anaemia progresses slowly, but the deterioration takes years
    C   eventually the treatment will cure the disease, and it can then be stopped
    D   the disease cannot be cured, but she will remain healthy with continuing treatment

Mark your answers here: 16.......17.......18.......19.......

16 D 69%

Pernicious anaemia results from inadequate absorption of vitamin B$_{12}$, associated with achlorhydria and deficiency of the intrinsic factor. A, B and C are all causes of other types of anaemia.

17 B 55%

Until Mrs Firth's haemoglobin rises above 7 g/100 ml she is at risk of developing heart failure if she exerts herself. The commode is less stressful than a bedpan.

18 A 90%

Schilling test measures the body's capacity to absorb vitamin B$_{12}$. B, C and D may all be performed, but will not identify the type of anaemia.

19 D 88%

Pernicious anaemia can be totally controlled with regular maintenance injections of Cobalomine, but it cannot be cured.

Eating and Drinking

Mrs Jenny Fiddler, a 23 year old barmaid, has been admitted to your ward at 6.00 am with a two day history of upper abdominal pain accompanied by vomiting. Her past history includes similar pains occurring at approximately five monthly intervals, lasting only 2-3 hours, with no vomiting. Jenny also states that fatty foods tend to disagree with her. A provisional diagnosis of acute pancreatitis is made.(RGN)

20 Which of the following investigations is most likely to assist the doctor to arrive at a diagnosis:

    A   assessing serum and urinary amylase levels
    B   taking a full blood count and haemoglobin level
    C   assessing serum and urinary glucose levels
    D   checking and monitoring temperature, pulse and blood pressure

21 Which of the following nursing actions will best help to reduce Jenny's symptoms:

    A   placing her in a sitting position
    B   administering intravenous glucose as prescribed
    C   withhold food and fluid by mouth
    D   pass a nasogastric tube and aspirate hourly

22 Which of the following treatments would be chosen when Jenny has been diagnosed as suffering from acute pancreatitis caused by a gall stone blocking the sphincter of Oddi:

    A   morphine 15 mg, prepantheline bromide four hourly and intravenous glucose
    B   pethidine 100 mg, diazepam 5 mg four hourly and intravenous dextrose
    C   diamorphine hydrochloride 10 mg, buscopan 20 mg and intravenous transfusion
    D   propantheline bromide 10 mg, pethidine 100 mg four hourly and intravenous saline

23 Which of the following actions must be undertaken in order to prevent recurrence of this condition in the future:

    A   control dietary intake of fat to the minimum
    B   advise the patient to avoid all dietary fat
    C   administration of prophylactic antibiotics
    D   exploratory surgery for removal of stones

Mark your answers here: 20.......21.......22.......23.......

20   A   59%

All of the investigations are necessary and have significance to pancreatitis but do not distinguish it from other abdominal conditions. Raised amylase levels are diagnostic with raised urinary amylase lasting for longer periods of time.

21   C   72%

Nothing is given by mouth as this would stimulate the pancreatic secretions and so exacerbate the condition.

22   D   36%

Propantheline bromide depresses vagal stimulation of pancreatic secretions. Pain is extremely severe, pethidine is most suitable as it reduces sphincter muscle spasm. Saline is necessary to maintain circulating fluid volume.

23   D   69%

The only action which can prevent recurrence is the removal of the stones.

Eating and Drinking

Mrs Shilton is a 43 year old lady who had a cholecystectomy and choledochotomy five days ago, and has been making a good recovery. Shortly after being visited by her husband and daughter, Mrs Shilton becomes anxious and asks to discharge herself.(RGN)

24 **The first course of action for the nurse in charge to take would be to**

A   advise Mrs Shilton of the consequences of her action
B   ask Mrs Shilton to sign the discharge form
C   try to contact Mrs Shilton's husband
D   try to discover the reason for Mrs Shilton's anxiety

25 **The most appropriate information to give Mrs Shilton before she goes home is that she should**

A   eat a normal diet
B   stay indoors for a week
C   eat a fat-free diet
D   contact her doctor immediately

26 **Which of the following would indicate that Mrs Shilton's 'T' tube can be removed:**

A   the drainage has stopped
B   it is the tenth postoperative day
C   she has no pain when the tube is clamped off
D   the cholangiogram shows the bile ducts are patent

Mark your answers here: 24.......25.......26.......

27

24   D   98%

The nurse might be able to relieve the anxiety, and Mrs Shilton might need to talk about her problems, think it over, and then come to a decision, instead of discharging herself on impulse; a course of action she might regret. Mrs Shilton may not want her husband to know she is upset.

25   A   63%

The reason for eating a fat-free diet has been removed. The hospital should inform Mrs Shilton's general practitioner of her discharge, and there is no special reason why she should stay indoors.

26   D   64%

The 'T' tube is inserted in the common bile duct at operation, and remains there until the danger of stricture formation is passed, about ten days after the operation. If the ducts are not patent then pain will be experienced when the tube is clamped, but the test to determine this is the 'T' tube cholangiogram, which is an objective way of discovering if strictures are present. Drainage will stop if the tube is not clamped, because the production of bile is continuous.

Mary, aged 2 years, is admitted for the repair of an umbilical hernia. Her mother is unable to be resident as she has a two month old baby. Mary and her mother visited the ward a week before admission.(RGN)

27 Which of the following types of behaviour would be considered normal in a two year old. To

A   play happily with others of a similar age
B   share most of his/her toys with others
C   readily accept strangers who are kind and gentle
D   be fearful of separation from parents

28 When admitting Mary the first priority of the nurse should be to

A   take a detailed nursing history from her mother before she leaves the ward
B   show a friendly and welcoming approach to Mary and her mother
C   ask her mother to sign the consent for the operation before she leaves
D   check that the details on Mary's identification band are correct

29 Mary is to be discharged the day after her operation. Which of the following should be the advice given to Mary's mother regarding care of Mary's wound:

A   bath her daily and allow the sutures to dissolve
B   keep her wound clean and dry, avoid Mary touching it
C   bathe her wound daily with cooled boiled water
D   keep her wound covered until she attends the outpatients department in 7 days time

30 On discharge Mary's mother should be warned that Mary is most likely to

A   have nightmares for a short while
B   regress a little in her behaviour
C   be very apprehensive about her wound site
D   demonstrate increased fear of strangers

Mark your answers here: 27.......28.......29.......30.......

27 D 91%

Two year olds are still very dependent, on their mother in particular, and cannot understand reasons for separation. Two year olds may play *alongside* others but they do not play together very much. They are still very possessive and have not yet learnt to share, and they are usually very shy.

28 B 93%

A friendly and welcoming approach to Mary and her mother will help to put both at ease and so help in building up a relationship. The nurse is not responsible for asking the mother to sign the consent form, this is the responsibility of the doctor. A and D are important but B should be the nurse's *first* priority.

29 B 72%

Mary's wound will heal more satisfactorily if kept clean and dry. She may be curious and play with her wound, therefore she needs to be distracted. A and C are not recommended as suitable care for such wounds and D is unnecessary. To keep a wound covered this long may also encourage infections.

30 B 66%

After hospitalization young children often regress a little and may resort to more babyish behaviour. A, C and D may occur and may depend on how she was cared for in hospital, whether her experience was a relatively happy one or a very traumatic one. B is the *most* likely situation to occur.

Pauline Graham, a 37 year old married woman with two children, is admitted to the ward with a diagnosis of iron deficiency anaemia. She is pale, lethargic, has a sore tongue and dysphagia.(RGN)

31 **Which of the following medications would be most likely to be prescribed for Mrs Graham as a long-term therapy:**

  A cyanocobalamin
  B ascorbic acid
  C ferrous sulphate
  D folic acid

32 **The most likely complications to occur with the administration of iron replacement therapy are**

  A skin rashes and mouth ulcers
  B constipation and intestinal irritation
  C dizziness and fainting
  D palpitation and tachycardia

33 **Which of the following techniques should be adopted for administration of an Inferon injection intramuscularly to avoid staining of Mrs Graham's skin:**

  A skin stretched tightly and needle inserted deeply into muscle
  B deep intramuscular injection and slow ejection of drugs into skin
  C massage skin to disperse depot of drug after administration
  D injection should be administered deeply into muscle using 'Z' injection technique

34 **Which of the following will best allay Mrs Graham's anxiety about her glossitis and dysphagia. Advise her that**

  A once her iron levels are restored the problems will resolve themselves
  B the glossitis and dysphagia will be with her permanently until the menopause is reached
  C they are not associated with the problems of iron deficiency
  D they are a result of bacteria which thrive in the absence of iron, and should therefore be resolved with treatment

Mark your answers here: 31........32........33........34.......

31 C 87%

Ferrous sulphate is an inexpensive iron preparation which will meet
Mrs Graham's needs when her acute anaemia has been treated.

32 B 94%

Constipation and gastrointestinal irritation occur because iron salts
are astringent. The reasons for constipation are not quite clear.

33 D 66%

'Z' injection technique prevents backflow of the solution into the
superficial layer of the skin, therefore preventing staining.

34 A 68%

Glossitis and dysphagia are symptoms of iron deficiency anaemia
and should resolve with treatment.

Simon aged 7 years is admitted to your ward with an acute intestinal obstruction. His mother accompanies him and is very distressed as Simon is anxious, pale and in pain.(RGN)

35 The reason why the doctor asks for a nasogastric tube to be passed soon after Simon's admission is in order to

A   prevent paralytic ileus
B   avoid further fluid loss
C   minimise vomiting
D   decrease peristaltic action

36 Simon goes to theatre where he is found to have a volvulus, 6 cm of gangrenous gut is resected. He returns to the ward, conscious but drowsy. Which of the following should be reported to the senior nurse immediately:

A   axillary temperature 36.2°C, pulse rate 110, respiratory rate 22
B   axillary temperature 38°C, pulse rate 130, respiratory rate 30
C   axillary temperature 37°C, pulse rate 94, respiratory rate 20
D   axillary temperature 36.7°C, pulse rate 150, respiratory rate 46

37 The doctor writes Simon up for an intramuscular injection of pethidine 10 mg. The ampoule contains 25 mg in 2 ml. The correct amount to be given will be

A   0.5 ml
B   0.6 ml
C   0.8 ml
D   1.2 ml

38 Which of the following is the reason for the drain which the doctor inserts into Simon's wound during the operation:

A   to detect any haemorrhage early
B   to detect any early infection
C   to prevent the formation of adhesions
D   to prevent the collection of an exudate

Mark your answers here: 35.......36.......37.......38.......

35   C   81%

A nasogastric tube will not prevent paralytic ileus, as it is usually the paralytic ileus that causes the vomiting. It cannot prevent the secretion of gastric and intestinal juices, so will not affect fluid loss, and it will have no effect on peristaltic action.

36   D   63%

The normal pulse rate and respiratory rate of a 7 year old, would be respectively, 80 to 90 and 18 to 24. Some rise is to be expected, but a pulse rate of 150 and respiratory rate of 46, with a normal temperature, is worrying.

37   C   86%

The formula for calculating paediatric drug dosages is

$$\frac{\text{what you want}}{\text{what you've got}} \times \text{the volume you've got it in.}$$

38   D   94%

If any exudate collects, there is more likely to be abscess formation, and healing will be delayed. If the drain was to detect haemorrhage, it could be removed after about 24 hours.

James Gill, aged seven years, has recently developed diabetes mellitus. He is admitted to a paediatric ward for stabilisation, and in order that he and his family can learn how to cope with his condition. James has a four year old sister.(RGN)

39   James' treatment will probably include

A   oral hypoglycaemic agents
B   subcutaneous insulin
C   intravenous insulin
D   oral insulin preparations

40   Which of the following is the most appropriate nursing response when James finds it hard to accept the necessary dietary restrictions, particularly when he sees his little sister eating sweets? To

A   relax diet restrictions as James is so young and hope he will adjust better in a year or two
B   suggest to James' parents that their daughter shares the same restricted diet as James
C   keep special treats like chocolate bars for occasions when swimming or football is played
D   tell James that he can only go home when he sticks to his diet all the time

41   Which of the following is the most appropriate nursing advice if James' mother is concerned about the cost of special diabetic foods:

A   these are essential to health and financial assistance may be available
B   these are non-essential and can be used just as treats to help James have variety
C   diabetic foods are necessary in order for diabetic children to feel 'normal'
D   these diabetic foods are intended primarily for adults and James should not have them

Mark your answers here: 39.......40.......41.......

39   B   82%

Oral insulin is destroyed by digestive enzymes. Oral hypoglycaemic agents are only useful for maturity onset diabetes.

40   C   60%

Mars bars etc. are useful carbohydrate boosters prior to strenuous exercise, and James will look forward to his 'treats'.

41   B   69%

Diabetic foods use sweeteners other than glucose, and can be used as *treats* for James. They are often used as convenience foods to add variety to the diet.

Gillian Lewis aged 19 years is an occupational therapy student and a newly diagnosed diabetic. She is attending outpatients in order to help her synchronise her diet and her insulin and to obtain good control of her blood sugar.(RGN)

42   **Gillian is planning to go to a party, and asks your advice about a special diabetic lager that she has seen.** The most appropriate comment is

A   not to drink alcohol at all as it will damage her arteries
B   that diabetic beers are more alcoholic than ordinary beers
C   to drink only fruit juice or mineral waters because they are low in carbohydrates
D   not to go to the party as it will interfere with achieving the balance between insulin and diet

43   **Which of the following is the most appropriate piece of advice when Gillian has been reluctant to give her own insulin but is now happy to do this into her left thigh; she prefers this site as it is easily accessible. To**

A   leave the situation as Gillian is giving her own insulin safely
B   tell Gillian that she must rotate injection sites whatever her own preference may be
C   discuss with Gillian the problems of insulin atrophy and the resulting poor diabetic control
D   arrange for a community nurse to give Gillian's insulin for a few days

44   **Gillian is worried about hypoglycaemic attacks that may happen when she is working as this could be dangerous for her patients.** The most effective way to help is to:

A   describe the onset of hypoglycaemic attacks to Gillian
B   advise her to keep in the 1-2% sugar range to prevent hypoglycaemic attacks
C   create the opportunity for Gillian to experience a hypoglycaemic attack
D   advise her to seek employment away from patient care

Mark your answers here: 42.......43.......44.......

42 B 52%

Diabetics should be warned about the high alcohol content of diabetic beers. As far as possible Gillian should lead a normal life.

43 C 62%

Once Gillian realises the possibility of scarring and the variable absorption of insulin if injected into one site she may accept the need for site rotation.

44 C 84%

By experiencing a hypoglycaemic attack Gillian can recognise the symptoms of onset and take action.

Jenny Reed, 20 years old, was admitted three days ago in a critical and drowsy state. She has been diagnosed as having insulin dependent diabetes mellitus. She is now much better and beginning to look after herself. She works as a shop assistant and plans to marry next year.(RGN)

45 Which of the following groups of clinical features were most likely to present when Jenny was admitted:

A weight gain, glycosuria, skin infections
B thirst, albuminuria, dehydration
C weight loss, glycosuria, thirst
D pruritus, nocturia, weight gain

46 Which of the following would have been the priority in Jenny's management on admission:

A restore fluids by encouraging intake of 3 litres daily
B lower blood glucose levels by insulin administration
C explain to her that she has diabetes
D ensure she is settled on the ward

47 Which of the following points must be emphasised when teaching Jenny about administration of insulin? She must:

A never omit her injections
B change the site of injections daily
C always cleanse the skin prior to injection
D have a main meal within thirty minutes

48 When Jenny asks you about her hopes of having a family you should

A advise her not to have a family as diabetes is hereditary
B tell her she can have a family as the risks are very slight
C suggest she makes an appointment to see a genetic counsellor when she goes home
D arrange for Jenny and her fiancé to see the consultant looking after her

Mark your answers here: 45.......46.......47.......48.......

45 C 80%

These symptoms are typical of a person with acute onset diabetes. Weight gain, skin infections and nocturia are typical of maturity onset, and albuminuria is a symptom of nephropathy.

46 B 90%

The critical condition is ketoacidosis leading to drowsiness, this can only be corrected by giving insulin so that cells can utilise glucose and thus stop the breakdown of proteins and fats. Fluids will be replaced as a priority but intravenously and in greater volume.

47 A 66%

All four are to some extent true. Injection sites should be used on a rotational basis, but not necessarily changed daily. Good hygiene is necessary but specific skin cleansing is not. Injections must be followed by food but not necessarily a main meal.

48 D 84%

There is a family tendency in diabetes, and both parties should have this explained to them.

Mrs Smith, a 60 year old housewife, is admitted to hospital for re-stabilisation of diabetes mellitus. She has had bilateral leg ulcers and bilateral cataracts for over two years. Until her admission, Mrs Smith looked after her severely crippled husband.(RGN)

49 Which of the following groups of clinical features is *most* likely to indicate that Mrs Smith's diabetes mellitus is out of control:

A repeated infections, constant tiredness, and excessive thirst
B repeated infections, cold extremities and genital pruritus
C genital pruritus, excessive thirst and cold extremities
D excessive thirst, constant headaches and genital pruritus

50 The best way to apply Mrs Smith's leg bandages is to start spiral bandaging from:

A behind the toe to below the knee
B above the ankle to below the knee
C below the ankle to below the knee
D above the ankle to above the knee

51 Which of the following should be the initial nursing action when Mrs Smith is found to have pyrexia, and *Clostridium welchii* in her wound swab:

A perform Mrs Smith's wound toilet three times daily
B ascertain that adequate antibiotics are given
C move Mrs Smith into a side ward or a quiet area of the ward
D perform Mrs Smith's wound toilet twice daily

52 The main reason why insulin is given by hypodermic injection to Mrs Smith is to

A promote a slow release
B aid rapid absorption and action
C prevent gastric impact
D avoid the digestive process

Mark your answers here: 49........50........51........52........

Answers

49 A 76%

Mrs Smith is most likely to complain of repeated infections, constant tiredness and excessive thirst. These symptoms are the first clinical features which are likely to appear in a diabetic patient.

50 A 80%

Spiral bandaging from behind the toes to below the knee is the best technique because it will allow drainage of peripheral fluids from the foot. The other bandaging techniques will cause congestion of fluid in the feet and toes.

51 C 52%

To prevent the spread of infection Mrs Smith would have to be isolated. The other nursing actions do not prevent infection spreading.

52 D 58%

Insulin is a protein and therefore it will be digested if it is given orally. Hypodermic injection does not aid rapid absorption action, therefore insulin should be given at least 30 minutes before the patient is given her food to allow absorption and readiness for action. If insulin is given too early without carbohydrate cover, the patient may develop hypoglycaemia.

2 : BREATHING

Mr Bernard Jason, a 47 year old car salesman, is admitted to your ward, suffering from a myocardial infarction. Mr Jason is of normal weight, but smokes 20 cigarettes per day, and remains very anxious during his stay in hospital. On admission he is attached to a cardiac monitor.(EN)

53 Which of the following would be the nurse's first action if she notices that the ECG trace on Mr Jason's monitor showed asystole:

    A   note Mr Jason's clinical condition
    B   call for assistance
    C   commence external cardiac massage
    D   prepare the defibrillator

54 Mr Jason states that he wants to stop smoking, which of the following is the most effective way to encourage him:

    A   tell him about the dangers of smoking
    B   frequently praise him for attempting to stop smoking
    C   ask his wife to bring sweets for him to suck
    D   search his locker daily for hidden cigarettes

55 Which of the following would be the most appropriate action when five days after admission, Mr Jason unsuccessfully tries to use the commode, and says he feels constipated:

    A   tell him not to worry, this is to be expected, but he should not strain
    B   offer him a strong laxative
    C   advise him to try again later
    D   suggest that you gently insert a suppository to help him

56 Mr Jason is prescribed glyceryl trinitrate. This drug is a

    A   beta blocker
    B   diuretic
    C   vasodilator
    D   sedative

Mark your answers here: 53.......54.......55.......56.......

53 A 67%

A common reason for the monitor showing a 'flat' trace is a fault with the electrodes, e.g. disconnection. Further action should not be taken until the nurse ascertains that Mr Jason has, in fact, suffered a cardiac arrest.

54 B 81%

Mr Jason needs people to encourage and support him in a positive way, and this is best accomplished by reinforcing his desire to stop smoking.

55 D 80%

A suppository would help Mr Jason to have his bowels opened with the minimum of effort, without the abdominal pain or diarrhoea which can accompany a strong laxative.

56 C 76%

Glyceryl trinitrate relieves angina pain by dilating the coronary arteries, thus increasing the blood supply to the myocardium.

Breathing

Mr Herbert Tinker is a 66 year old man who suffers from chronic bronchitis and has now developed heart failure for which he has been admitted to hospital.(EN)

57 Which of the following signs will the nurse expect to find in the admission assessment:

A exhaustion, bruising, dyspnoea
B bruising, dyspnoea, oedema
C dyspnoea, oedema, exhaustion
D oedema, exhaustion, bruising

58 When observing Mr Tinker's apex beat and pulse, which of the following would the nurse expect to find? Apex beat

A strong and regular, pulse rate regular and weak
B strong and regular, pulse rate irregular and weak
C weak and rapid, pulse rate regular and weak
D weak and rapid, pulse rate irregular and weak

59 The best explanation to give Mr Tinker about his daily weighing is that it is to

A check that he has sufficient fluid intake
B monitor his weight loss due to anorexia
C monitor the effectiveness of his diuretic therapy
D check that he is eating the correct amount

60 Which of the following is the correct explanation for Mr Tinker's loss of energy:

A his recent inability to eat an adequate diet
B his heart is unable to supply his body cells with sufficient oxygen
C muscle wasting resulting from his inability to exercise
D loss of taste and halitosis because of infected sputum

Mark your answers here: 57.......58.......59.......60.......

57   C   69%

These result from poor circulation and oxygenation caused by poor heart action and lung congestion.

58   D   60%

Heart failure produces weak ineffective heart action resulting in lost beats in the periphery which are felt as a weak and irregular pulse.

59   C   81%

Weighing is the most accurate record of fluid loss as 1 litre of water weighs 1 kg.

60   B   80%

Poor oxygenation means insufficient oxygen supply to the muscles and also causes poor digestion and therefore lack of nutrients to tissues.

Whilst walking through the park you are asked by a young boy to look at his friend who is unwell. 5 year old Timothy is laying on a bench and is suffering from epistaxis.(EN)

61   Which of the following first aid measures would you take:

    A   sit him up with his head forward and nose pinched
    B   lay him down in the recovery position and pinch his nose
    C   sit him up with his head back and nose pinched
    D   lay him down, elevate his legs, and pinch his nose

62   The reason for pinching his nose is because

    A   indirect pressure promotes haemostasis
    B   swallowing is prevented
    C   nose breathing is prevented
    D   direct pressure promotes haemostasis

63   Which would you do when the bleeding stops:

    A   send the boys to get some ice
    B   send the other boy away
    C   send one boy to summon Timothy's parents
    D   send one boy to find a doctor

Mark your answers here: 61.......62.......63.......

61   A   82%

Sitting up with his head forward allows blood to run out, rather than being swallowed or inhaled.

62   D   84%

Pinching the nose puts direct pressure on the bleeding point which slows the blood flow and promotes clotting.

63   C   86%

Your first aid measures have been successful, further action should be under parental control.

Mr Allen, a 60 year old retired miner who has been a heavy smoker for many years, is admitted to your ward with an exacerbation of his chronic obstructive airways disease. He has a bubbly cough, is extremely breathless and agitated. He is also overweight.(EN)

64 Which of the following types of masks would be best used when giving prescribed oxygen therapy to Mr Allen:

A nasal cannulae
B Hudson mask
C ventimask
D oxygen tent

65 The reason why Mr Allen should have 24-28% oxygen is

A to counteract the high level of carbon dioxide in his blood
B because hypoxia has become the principal respiratory drive
C because he is likely to be on continuous oxygen therapy
D because of his reduced respiratory rate

66 The best combination of nursing actions to relieve Mr Allen's dyspnoea is

A to encourage mobility and weigh daily
B to administer prescribed bronchial dilators
C oxygen therapy, bed-rest
D to administer prescribed diuretics

67 The most common complication of chronic obstructive airways disease is

A myocardial infarction
B tuberculosis
C hypertension
D cor pulmonale

Mark your answers here: 64.......65.......66.......67.......

Answers

64 C 64%

A ventimask should be used when accurate percentages of oxygen are needed especially low concentrations in chronic obstructive airways disease.

65 B 57%

Carbon dioxide is the normal respiratory stimulant. Over a period of time the respiratory centre adapts to the hypoxic situation. Therefore a high concentration of oxygen may depress respiration.

66 C 58%

This combination increases the oxygen available to Mr Allan at the same time decreasing his demand for oxygen. Together these relieve his dyspnoea.

67 D 67%

Cor pulmonale is right-sided heart failure secondary to chronic obstructive airways disease, which increases the workload of the right side of the heart, and therefore is common with chronic obstructive airway disease.

Mrs Joan Brown, a 27 year old housewife, and mother of two young children, is admitted to a medical ward with severe right-sided chest pain and breathlessness. Until this occasion she has been fairly fit with no previous relevant history. The patient is anxious, and a provisional diagnosis of spontaneous pneumothorax is made.(EN)

68 The term pneumothorax is best described as

    A   pus in the pleural cavity
    B   air in the pleural cavity
    C   pus outside the pleural cavity
    D   air outside the pleural cavity

69 Which of the following would be the most important reason for inserting an underwater seal drain into Mrs Brown's chest:

    A   to reduce the risk of complications
    B   to allow excess air to escape from the lungs
    C   to regain negative pressure inside the pleural sac
    D   to prevent further air from entering the pleural sac

70 During routine nursing care the underwater seal drainage bottle is accidently knocked over. The nurse's first action should be to

    A   place the bottle upright
    B   check the system for damage
    C   check the 'swing' in the tube
    D   clamp the tube

71 Which of the following is the reason why the underwater seal drainage tubing should be clamped prior to moving Mrs Brown:

    A   to make Mrs Brown more comfortable
    B   to prevent fluid from the bottle syphoning into Mrs Brown's chest
    C   to allow the drain to continue functioning correctly
    D   to ensure that excess air does not leak from Mrs Brown's lungs to the bottle

Mark your answers here: 68.......69.......70.......71.......

68   B   92%

Air in the pleural cavity caused as a result of perforation of the chest wall or lung pleura.

69   C   46%

Under normal circumstances there is a slight negative pressure between the layers of the pleura. This ensures expansion of the lungs during inspiration. When all the air is removed, and no more enters the pleural sac the negative pressure will be restored.

70   D   64%

This would prevent air from entering the pleural cavity. Once checks are made for damage, observation of the *swing* in the tube could then be carried out.

71   B   88%

If the drainage bottle is lifted above the level of Mrs Brown's chest, there is a danger that fluid will syphon into her chest if the tube is not changed.

James, aged 3 years, is admitted to your ward during an acute asthmatic attack. He is a known asthmatic, but has not previously required hospital admission. James, who is an only child, and is very wheezy and distressed, is accompanied by his mother.(RGN)

72   Which of the following best describes the condition of James' lungs during an acute asthmatic attack:

    A   bronchospasm and an excessive production of frothy white sputum
    B   inflammation of the mucous membranes and collapse of the alveoli
    C   an excessive production of thick viscid mucus and bronchospasm
    D   productive cough and inflammation of the mucous membranes

73   Which of the following statements is true:

    A   alveolar resistance is decreased
    B   residual volume is increased
    C   tidal volume is increased
    D   dead space air is decreased

74   The signs and symptoms that James will most likely suffer from during the attack are

    A   an inspiratory stridor and barrel chest
    B   an expiratory wheeze and hoarse cry
    C   an intercostal recession and expiratory wheeze
    D   a paroxysmal cough and inspiratory stridor

75   James' restless condition shortly after admission is due to

    A   hypercapnia
    B   hypoxia
    C   acidosis
    D   dehydration

Mark your answers here: 72....... 73....... 74....... 75.......

72 C 69%

During an asthmatic attack there is spasm of the bronchial muscles, inflammation of the mucous membranes lining the tract, and an increase in the production of thick sticky mucus. Sometimes there is a cough, but it is non-productive as the secretions are too thick to be removed. The alveoli become overdistended, they do not collapse.

73 B 64%

The narrowing of the airways causes overinflation of the lungs, as expiration is more difficult than inspiration. The alveolar resistance and residual volume are both increased. The tidal volume is decreased. The dead space air is unaltered.

74 C 62%

James is likely to have an expiratory wheeze, and intercostal recession due to his difficulty in breathing. He may have a paroxysmal cough, and may be barrel chested due to the overinflation of the lungs. An inspiratory stridor and hoarse cry are more likely to occur in croup, where there is obstruction to the upper airways and difficulty in inspiration.

75 B 64%

Lack of oxygen to the brain cells causes restlessness and possibly disorientation. Hypercapnia causes apathy and exhaustion. Acidosis causes headache and drowsiness. Dehydration causes apathy and coma may eventually occur.

Kathy Coles, a sixteen year old schoolgirl studying for her 'O' levels, is admitted to the Accident and Emergency Department. Kathy has been a known asthmatic since she was seven years old, and is now diagnosed as having status asthmaticus.(RGN)

76 **A definition of status asthmaticus is**

A   difficulty in breathing for several hours
B   wheezing with expiratory dyspnoea over a prolonged period of time
C   an imbalance in respiratory function causing difficulty in breathing
D   respiratory embarrassment on inspiration

77 **Which of the following combinations of drug therapy is most likely to be prescribed for immediate administration in the Accident and Emergency Department:**

A   intravenous aminophylline and intravenous hydrocortisone
B   salbutamol and Intal inhalation
C   aminophylline suppositories and oral salbutamol
D   diazepam, salbutamol and prednisolone orally

78 **The most likely precipitating factor in Kathy's present attack is**

A   an allergic reaction
B   excessive physical exercise
C   worry about her examinations
D   consumption of a heavy meal

79 **In assessing respiratory function a peak flow meter is used. This measures**

A   the forced expiratory volume
B   vital capacity
C   tidal volume
D   residual volume

Mark your answers here: 76.......77.......78.......79.......

76 B 85%

Prolonged and intractable asthma is referred to as 'status asthmaticus' and the main problem with asthma is one of expiration, because of spasm of the bronchioles.

77 A 86%

Intravenous aminophylline 250 mg will produce immediate partial relief from distress. Intravenous hydrocortisone 100 mg should be given as soon as possible, the main management being based on giving large doses of corticosteroids and ensuring adequate oxygenation.

78 C 89%

Though all are possible precipitating factors, the most likely in Kathy's case is her anxiety over GCE examinations.

79 A 80%

Measures the forced expiratory volume which is reduced in asthma and other forms of bronchoconstriction.

Jane is thirty-five years old and she is suffering from left-sided heart failure caused by mitral stenosis. She has five year old twins and lives alone with them in a damp basement flat. She is admitted to a medical ward for assessment. (RGN)

80   Jane is suffering from dyspnoea because of

    A   reduced air intake to lungs
    B   lack of haemoglobin in blood
    C   increased pressure in the left atrium
    D   increased cardiac output

81   Which of the following combinations of drugs will Jane be most likely to be given:

    A   indomethacin, potassium chloride, digoxin, frusemide
    B   digoxin, potassium chloride, frusemide, heparin
    C   digoxin, amoxycillin, potassium chloride, heparin
    D   indomethacin, digoxin, heparin, frusemide

82   Which of the following should Jane be given before she is discharged home:

    A   information about medication, an exercise programme, discussion of possible future surgery, social services support
    B   dietary advice, information about medication, advice to rest for long periods, ways of coping with chronic illness
    C   information about medication, discussion of possible future surgery, dietary advice, social services support
    D   ways of coping with chronic illness, advice to rest for long periods, social services support

Mark your answers here: 80.......81.......82.......

80 C 72%

Jane's mitral stenosis will cause problems with left ventricular filling, giving rise to increased left atrial pressure, and back-pressure in the lungs, causing pulmonary oedema.

81 B 54%

Digoxin will control the heart beat, frusemide and potassium chloride will prevent or treat pulmonary oedema, and heparin will prevent clots forming round the diseased valve.

82 C 42%

Jane is a probable candidate for valve replacement in the future and social services may help her to cope until this is possible. She should avoid obesity, and needs advice about her medication.

Breathing

Mrs Florence Mayes, aged 62, is admitted with cor pulmonale. She presents with dyspnoea and oedema.(RGN)

83   The best description of cor pulmonale is

    A   left-sided heart failure secondary to right-sided heart failure
    B   disease of the lungs secondary to left-sided heart failure
    C   right-sided heart failure secondary to pulmonary disease
    D   disease of the lungs secondary to right-sided heart failure

84   The cause of Mrs Mayes' oedema is

    A   loss of protein in her urine
    B   increased renin production by the kidneys
    C   increased venous hydrostatic pressure
    D   decreased circulation of blood to the lungs

85   Mrs Mayes is prescribed salbutamol via a patient triggered ventilator. The correct way for Mrs Mayes to use the machine is

    A   to breathe out before inspiring when using the machine
    B   to exhale forcefully into the machine and then to breathe normally
    C   to inhale as deeply as she can and to blow all the air out into the machine
    D   to breathe in through her nose and exhale into the machine

Mark your answers here: 83.......84.......85.......

83   C   80%

It is the only one which is correct, as cor pulmonale means heart disease which is secondary to lung disease.

84   C   64%

Increased pressure in the venous capillaries, caused by back pressure from the heart, would prevent fluid re-entering the circulation thereby causing oedema.

85   A   92%

It is important to empty the lungs before using the ventilator to allow for maximum inflation.

Mrs Jones, aged 75 years, is admitted to the medical ward at 02.00 hours. She is dyspnoeic, confused, cyanosed and cold. Mrs Jones is widowed, lives alone and is very independent. A diagnosis of heart failure is made.(RGN)

86 Relief of the following problems requires immediate management on admission:

    A cyanosis
    B confusion
    C dyspnoea
    D anxiety

87 Which of the following drugs could be used to relieve bronchial constriction and act as a diuretic:

    A frusemide
    B aminophylline
    C Moduretic
    D salbutamol

88 Which action should be taken if Mrs Jones becomes more confused during the night:

    A give her a prescribed dose of sedatives
    B sit with her and try to reassure her
    C put up cot sides and give prescribed medication
    D give high concentration of oxygen to relieve anoxia

89 The best way to help Mrs Jones' temperature to return to normal is to

    A use a 'space blanket'
    B wrap Mrs Jones in extra blankets
    C nurse Mrs Jones near a radiator
    D allow her to 'warm up' as treatment takes effect

Mark your answers here: 86.......87.......88.......89.......

86   C   92%

Relief of dyspnoea is most important, it will reduce respiratory effort and therefore anxiety. Reduction of dyspnoea, and better respiratory intake of oxygen, increases oxygen levels in the blood thereby relieving cerebral anoxia and therefore confusion.

87   B   56%

Aminophylline reduces bronchial constriction and has a mild diuretic effect, these actions combine to reduce pulmonary oedema.

88   B   76%

The most appropriate action would be to stay with her and try reassuring her. Mild sedatives and cot sides may be given and used. If sedated, Mrs Jones may lose the anoxic drive. Cot sides increase the feeling of being trapped. A high concentration of oxygen increases O_2 levels and reduces anoxic drive.

89   A   76%

Space blankets conserve the patient's body heat, thus raising the temperature slowly. This is the preferred treatment for hypothermia.

Jenny, aged four months, is admitted to your ward because of severe coughing attacks, which are diagnosed as pertussis (whooping cough). Prior to admission a cubicle is prepared for her arrival. Jenny is found to have moderately severe paroxysmal coughing attacks.(RGN)

90 Which of the following is the most appropriate for Jenny. A cubicle containing

A   a gown, mask and a warm environment
B   an incubator, oxygen and intravenous infusion equipment
C   oxygen, suction and a cool environment
D   intravenous infusion equipment, oxygen tent and humidity

91 When Jenny has a coughing attack the most important action is to

A   maintain an adequate airway
B   prevent vomiting
C   comfort the baby
D   provide adequate hydration

92 Which of the following 'milestones' should Jenny be able to achieve:

A   rest on forearms and hold head up when in prone position
B   transfer objects from one hand to another
C   discriminate between strangers and close members of the family
D   drop toys over the side of the cot

93 Which of the following must the mother be asked about before her child is vaccinated against pertussis for the first time. If the child has had

A   asthma
B   convulsions
C   eczema
D   jaundice

Mark your answers here: 90.......91.......92.......93.......

90   C   50%

The reason being that babies with whooping cough have a pyrexia, and therefore require a cool environment. Because of the paroxysmal attacks, suction and oxygen may be required. An intravenous infusion would not be needed in an uncomplicated attack of pertussis.

91   A   86%

The most important action here is to maintain a clear airway by removing nasal and oral secretion and any vomit which occurs.

92   A   82%

At four months old Jenny will have gained some head control therefore she can hold her head up in the prone position. The other achievements are not usually developed until a child is approximately six to nine months, though one has to remember that there are great variations on normal.

93   B   72%

In 1981 the DHSS published the conclusions of a report stating that pertussis vaccinations should not be carried out if the child has a history of convulsions, cerebral irritation or damage in the neonatal period. This was to safeguard against any possible reactions to whooping cough vaccine.

Paul Daniels, the manager of a small engineering firm, is admitted to the ward following retrosternal chest pain radiating down his left arm. He is pale, anxious, and obviously in pain. A diagnosis of myocardial infarction is made.(RGN)

94 Which of the following should be a priority of care on admission:

    A relief of anxiety
    B monitoring vital signs
    C relief of pain
    D relief of nausea

95 Which of the following cardiac arrhythmias would give most concern if it appears on Mr Daniels' cardiac monitor:

    A atrial fibrillation
    B ventricular fibrillation
    C ventricular ectopic
    D sinus arrhythmia

96 The reason why you would allow Mr Daniels to use the commode rather than the bed pan is because the use of the commode

    A increases oxygen demand to the heart
    B reduces blood flow to the heart
    C makes it easier to move the patient if arrest occurs
    D is less exertive and places less strain on the heart

97 The most likely complication of myocardial infarction is

    A right ventricular failure
    B left ventricular failure
    C mitral valve stenosis
    D congestive heart failure

Mark your answers here: 94.......95.......96.......97.......

94   C   75%

Relief of pain is most important since by doing this anxiety and nausea will be reduced.

95   B   81%

Mr Daniels' cardiac output, and heart rate will be incompatible with life.

96   D   96%

Use of the commode is less tiring and more comfortable for the patient, it therefore reduces anxiety and strain.

97   B   49%

If a large area of the left ventricle's myocardium is deprived of it's blood supply, the rest of the myocardium has to work harder to maintain cardiac output, and may fail.

Breathing

Mr Andrew Barkby, a 63 year old businessman, is admitted to your ward for the insertion of a permanent pacemaker, following several Stokes-Adams attacks. Mr Barkby is accompanied by his wife who is just about to leave the ward when Mr Barkby has a cardiac arrest.(RGN)

98 Which of the following would indicate that a cardiac arrest has occurred:

A unconscious with fixed dilated pupils
B no carotid pulse and unconscious
C cyanosed with no respirations
D fixed dilated pupils and cyanosed

99 The most accurate description of a classical Stokes-Adams attack is that

A the patient stops breathing and goes blue
B it is similar to an asthmatic attack but more serious
C the patient has a mild epileptiform fit
D it is similar to a cardiac arrest but with spontaneous recovery

100 Which of the following is most important for Mr Barkby to perform regularly when he leaves hospital:

A feel the pacemaker under his skin
B check his pulse
C perform a set exercise regime
D record his temperature

101 Which of the following is the type of pacemaker Mr Barkby will probably have fitted:

A internal, demand
B external, demand
C internal, fixed rate
D external, fixed rate

Mark your answers here: 98.......99.......100.......101.......

67

Answers

98 B 88%

The carotid pulse would be absent because Mr Barkby's heart has stopped, and cerebral anoxia would lead to unconsciousness. Fixed dilated pupils and absence of respiration would follow.

99 D 85%

Stokes-Adams attacks are caused by short periods of asystole from which the heart recovers spontaneously. This means that the patient will appear to have a cardiac arrest as the cardiac output falls.

100 B 58%

If Mr Barkby's pulse is outside limits set by the doctors it may mean that the pacemaker has failed. This necessitates urgent medical attention.

101 A 55%

Most permanent pacemakers are internal, inserted under the skin of the chest wall. They are usually set only to generate impulses if the patient's own heart rate falls below a set rate (demand).

68

3 : MOBILISING

Mrs Brown, a 67 year old widow, has had rheumatoid arthritis for several years resulting in a number of hospital admissions. She has been re-admitted for arthrodesis of her left knee.(EN)

102　Which of the following statements is true? Rheumatoid arthritis:

    A   is more common in men than women
    B   only affects the middle-aged and elderly
    C   is equally common in men and women
    D   affects all age groups

103　Which of the following actions will Mrs Brown find most difficult in the early post-operative days:

    A   rising from a chair to stand
    B   standing for a few minutes
    C   turning over in bed
    D   walking

104　Which of the following actions will Mrs Brown be unable to perform independently when she goes home with the necessary aids:

    A   putting on her shoes
    B   cutting her toe nails
    D   using the toilet
    D   washing her legs

Mark your answers here: 102.......103.......104.......

102 D 68%

Rheumatoid arthritis affects all age groups, even though the onset often occurs in young adults.

103 A 66%

Mrs Brown's stiff knee would cause particular difficulties when getting out of a chair.

104 B 80%

Aids will allow Mrs Brown a great deal of independence, but she will not be able to reach her toes to cut her nails.

Mrs Annie Smithson, an active 73 year old lady is admitted to your ward having sustained a transcervical fracture of the left femur in a fall at home. Mrs Smithson lives with her fit 75 year old husband, and has two daughters who live nearby. She is a very popular lady with many friends in the local community.(EN)

105 Which of the following contributes to the fact that more old ladies suffer this injury than old gentlemen:

    A   old ladies are generally more active than old men
    B   osteoporosis, a predisposing factor, is more common in women
    C   old ladies tend to have poor eyesight, and trip over rugs etc.
    D   there are more old ladies in the population than old men

106 Mrs Smithson becomes mildly confused about time and place at night. The best way to minimise this is to

    A   leave a light by her bed so Mrs Smithson can see where she is
    B   agree with her, when Mrs Smithson says she is somewhere else
    C   frequently remind the patient where she is, and what the time is
    D   tell the patient that everything will be all right in the morning

107 Which of the following may develop if Mrs Smithson is not carefully supervised when she begins to mobilise after the operation:

    A   incontinence
    B   chest infection
    C   deep vein thrombosis
    D   dislocation of the prosthesis

Mark your answers here: 105.......106.......107.......

Answers

105 B 76%

One of the causes of osteoporosis is lack of the female hormone oestrogen, after the menopause. Oestrogen helps to maintain calcium in the bones, thus preventing osteoporosis.

106 C 78%

Mrs Smithson is probably confused because of the change of environment. If she is reminded about her environment she is more likely to remember what has happened to her, and be less confused.

107 D 96%

Dislocation of the prosthesis is the main danger at this point. The others are all complications of bed rest, not related to Mrs Smithson beginning to mobilise.

Mr Turner is 65 years old and recently retired. He lives with his wife in a bungalow on the edge of town. He has been admitted for assessment as he has recently been diagnosed as suffering from Parkinson's disease.(EN)

108 Which of the following would help confirm the diagnosis of Mr Turner's illness:

    A   a left hemiplegia
    B   muscle rigidity which can be seen in his mask-like facial expression
    C   generalised muscle weakness and flaccidity
    D   occasional bouts of muscle spasm

109 The best way for a newly qualified enrolled nurse to help Mr and Mrs Turner begin to come to terms with the disease is for her to

    A   explain the cause of the disease
    B   listen to their worries before asking a senior nurse to help if necessary
    C   arrange for them to talk to other patients with similar conditions
    D   point out other patients in the ward who are far more handicapped

110 Which of the following drugs will be most likely to be prescribed for Mr Turner:

    A   anticonvulsants to reduce muscle twitching
    B   anticoagulants to prevent thrombosis caused by reduced mobility
    C   L-dopa drugs to replace dopamine in the brain cells
    D   antidepressants to raise his mood

111 Which of the following services will provide the support Mr and Mrs Turner will need at home:

    A   the community nurse who visits daily
    B   meals on wheels
    C   a voluntary visitor to call each day
    D   the occupational therapist to assess the facilities at home

Mark your answers here: 108.......109.......110.......111.......

108 B 50%

One of Mr Turner's main problems is muscle rigidity which results in
a mask-like facial expression which causes family and friends to think
he is miserable or uninterested.

109 B 54%

As an enrolled nurse you will not be in the position to answer all Mr
and Mrs Turner's queries or to provide all the information they will
need, but your caring unhurried approach can elicit problems and
then, with the patient's agreement you can bring them to the attention
of the senior nurse.

110 C 70%

The exact cause of Parkinson's disease is not known but a reduction
of dopamine in certain brain cells has been found to cause muscle
rigidity, therefore medication with dopamine has proved to be
beneficial.

111 D 82%

The occupational therapist will visit the couple at home and assess
their needs. She can then arrange for appropriate action based on her
assessment.

John is a long distance lorry driver who has a long history of backache with pain radiating down his left leg. He is unmarried and lives in various digs around the country. He has been admitted for investigations and bed rest. The provisional diagnosis is prolapsed intervertebral disc.(EN)

112 The most appropriate position in which to nurse John is

A flat on a firm bed
B sitting up supported by strong backrest
C semi-prone supported by pillows
D prone

113 During his first few days in hospital John is most likely to complain of

A hunger and anxiety
B backache and constipation
C problems of elimination and backache
D weight loss and anorexia

114 Which of the following is it most important for John to learn before he is discharged from hospital:

A to take his drugs regularly
B how to lift properly
C how to choose the correct diet
D how to exercise efficiently

Mark your answers here: 112.......113.......114.......

Answers

112 A 90%

A firm bed will provide the necessary support while resting flat and will reduce the work demanded of the back muscles while the acute inflammation resolves.

113 C 86%

John will probably complain of backache from his disc. He may have difficulty passing urine or having his bowels opened in the hospital environment, especially if nursed flat.

114 B 86%

All aspects are important for patient health education but bearing in mind John's injury and occupation it is essential that he learns how to lift properly.

Mary is a 25 year old typist engaged to be married soon. Last week she had numbness in her right leg and yesterday her vision became blurred and she found that she had weakness in her left hand. She has been admitted for assessment with the diagnosis of multiple sclerosis.(EN)

115 Which of the following is the correct information to give Mary and her fiancé when they ask if the disease will be transmitted to their children:

A   that the disease is not hereditary so there is no risk to the next generation

B   the disease is unusual and therefore not likely to affect any babies they may have

C   that they should not have any children because of the high risk to the next generation

D   the disease is not hereditary but blood relatives are 10-15 times more likely to develop it than the rest of the population

116 Which of the following life styles should Mary be encouraged to follow:

A   as independent and active as she can be
B   restful, leading a quiet life
C   enjoy a strenuous life style
D   planning for a future spent in a wheelchair

117 The best way to evaluate Mary's condition is to

A   read through the care plan and check with the junior nurse that all the care has been given

B   look at Mary's observations and neurological assessment

C   ask sister or staff nurse to appraise your work

D   discuss with Mary whether the nursing care planned met her needs, and whether she has any fresh problems

Mark your answers here: 115.......116.......117.......

115 D 68%

As the cause of multiple sclerosis is not known it is difficult to be specific, but there is clear evidence that there is an increased risk in blood relatives, though there is no evidence of a hereditary factor.

116 A 98%

Multiple sclerosis is characterised by periods of remission, so that for several years Mary may be fit and well. She may even find that the disease stops totally, and she may always remain fairly fit.

117 D 86%

All the aspects mentioned are important, but as it is an evaluation of the care Mary has received, it is essential that she is involved in this process.

Mr John Grimson is a forty year old window cleaner. He has recently been complaining of pain in his legs when climbing his ladder, the pain is relieved by rest. He has also lost some feeling in his feet. John is subsequently admitted to your ward to have an arteriogram, when he is diagnosed as suffering from intermittent claudication.(RGN)

118 Which of the following is the cause of intermittent claudication:

    A   reduction of metabolic wastes in the muscles
    B   excessive demand of the tissues for oxygen
    C   abnormal metabolic process due to lack of oxygen
    D   inability of the muscles to metabolise oxygen

119 The reason why John has a bilateral aorto-femoral by-pass graft performed is in order to

    A   remove the obstruction in the artery
    B   by-pass the obstruction in the artery
    C   prevent the obstruction from worsening
    D   remove the obstruction to venous return

120 Which of the following aspects of John's life style may need changing if he is to enjoy good health after the operation:

    A   alcohol, smoking, exercise, diet
    B   smoking, exercise, diet, pedicure
    C   alcohol, smoking, exercise, pedicure
    D   alcohol, pedicure, diet, exercise

121 The reason why John is prescribed dipyridamole to take at home is in order to

    A   reduce the stickiness of platelets and dilate arteries
    B   vasodilate the veins and improve venous return
    C   thin the blood by reducing the clotting factors
    D   improve peripheral blood supply by increasing blood volume

Mark your answers here: 118.......119.......120.......121.......

118 C 56%

Oxygen lack to the tissues is caused by poor blood supply. Metabolites such as lactic acid are formed as a result of anaerobic metabolism, thus causing pain.

119 B 90%

This operation by passes the obstruction.

120 B 52%

Alcohol is not thought to contribute to atheroma, which caused John's condition. Smoking, a diet high in saturated fats, and lack of exercise, contribute to this condition.

121 A 50%

John may develop a blood clot at the site of operation. Dipyridamole is a safer way of preventing this than anticoagulants.

Alan Jones, aged **64** years, is a postman who has been diabetic for approximately twenty years. He had his left great toe amputated about ten months ago and has now been admitted to hospital because he has a gangrenous area on his right heel.(RGN)

122 Which of the following is the most likely cause of Alan's complaint that his left calf is painful when he has walked a few yards:

    A   muscular fatigue caused by exercise
    B   build up of toxic wastes in the tissue
    C   referred pain from the damaged heel
    D   imbalanced posture since his amputation

123 Which of the following should be the nurse's response when Alan says that he 'juggles' his insulin to suit his shifts at work, but his urine usually contains 1% sugar? She should:

    A   not intervene in Alan's routine as an established diabetic
    B   discuss this information with the doctor because it is vital to help Alan to achieve better control
    C   closely observe the degree of blood sugar control during Alan's stay in hospital
    D   take no action because blood sugar control is the doctor's concern

124 The best description of 'sliding scale insulin' is

    A   a gradually increasing dose of insulin
    B   a gradually decreasing dose of insulin
    C   a fluctuating dose of insulin
    D   a constant dose of insulin

125 Which of the following is most important when applying eusol and paraffin gauze to Alan's heel:

    A   have the solution at room temperature
    B   ensure that the gauze is thoroughly soaked
    C   apply the solution only to the necrotic area
    D   change the dressing every eight hours

Mark your answers here: 122.......123.......124.......125.......

122 B   45%

The pain described is intermittent claudication. It is caused by the build-up of toxic wastes resulting from abnormal metabolism in the cell in response to oxygen deprivation. The oxygen deprivation is due to impaired arterial blood flow.

123 B   77%

Blood sugar control is essential if Alan is to avoid amputation of his legs.

124 C   71%

The dose is calculated in response to urine or blood sugar levels.

125 C   87%

Eusol and paraffin will damage healthy skin.

Cynthia, a 19 year old single girl, is admitted to the medical ward with a diagnosis of deep vein thrombosis. She smokes 20-30 cigarettes daily and is on the contraceptive pill. Cynthia is prescribed intravenous heparin, to be given concurrently with oral warfarin for three days.(RGN)

126 **Which of the following would indicate an overdosage of anticoagulant:**

    A   coughing up blood stained sputum
    B   increasing tenderness of the calves of her legs
    C   sudden bleeding from the nose
    D   voiding of concentrated dark urine

127 **The antidote to heparin is**

    A   protamine sulphate
    B   vitamin K
    C   ferrous sulphate
    D   Dindevan

128 **If an embolus is dislodged from the thrombus in the leg, it is most likely to reach the lung via one of the following blood vessels:**

    A   superior vena cava
    B   pulmonary veins
    C   pulmonary artery
    D   jugular vein

129 **Which of the following should be reported immediately if seen in Cynthia:**

    A   haemoptysis
    B   pyrexia
    C   hypertension
    D   tachycardia

Mark your answers here: 126.......127.......128.......129.......

Answers

126 C 54%

Coughing up blood stained sputum may indicate a small pulmonary embolism, but sudden and unexplained epistaxis is most likely to be indicative of a heparin overdose.

127 A 86%

Protamine sulphate.

128 C 83%

Pulmonary artery, via the inferior vena cava, right atrium and right ventricle.

129 A 83%

Haemoptysis should be reported immediately as it may indicate pulmonary embolism.

Mrs Smythe is 74 years old. Until now, she has been an active independent lady, well able to look after herself. She has a history of mitral stenosis and today collapsed suddenly whilst cooking. She has been admitted unconscious with a left-sided hemiplegia and has been diagnosed as having had a stroke. Her daughter has accompanied her.(RGN)

130 Mrs Smythe will probably receive the following scores on the Norton scale:

A 7-10
B 10-12
C 12-14
D 14-16

131 Which of the following actions would you take when sitting Mrs Smythe out of bed 3 days after admission:

A her table on the left
B her table on the right
C in a chair with a fixed table
D no table but a bell in her right hand

132 Mrs Smythe cannot speak her words properly although she knows what she wants to say. Which one of the following describes this symptom:

A dysphagia
B dysphasia
C dysarthria
D dyslexia

133 Which of the following complications is Mrs Smythe most likely to develop in the initial stages of her illness:

A pressure sores
B urinary retention
C chest infection
D deep vein thrombosis

Mark your answers here: 130.......131.......132.......133.......

130 A   60%

A	physical condition	fair-good	3-4
B	neural condition	stuperous	1
C	activity	bedfast	1
D	mobility	immobile	1
E	incontinent	urine or double	1-2
		total	7-10

131 A   56%

If the things that Mrs Smythe needs are on her left side (her affected side) she must either learn to use her left hand or lean over with her right hand. This will also help her to become aware of her affected side, which she may ignore.

132 B   76%

Dysphagia means difficulty in swallowing, dysarthria means difficulty in articulation, dyslexia means difficulty in reading ability and dysphasia means incomplete language function and assembly of words associated with damage to the speech centre.

133 C   52%

Chest infection has the most rapid onset of the four. Organisms are already present in the respiratory tract and a lost or diminished cough reflex precipitates infection.

Miss Thomas, aged 74 years, is admitted for re-assessment of arthritis. She walks slowly with a stick and is independent in most tasks. Following her first night in hospital you observe her trying to conceal a wet nightdress. She looks upset and tries to hurry to the bathroom. Her nursing assessment did not reveal any incontinence.(RGN)

134   The nurse's choice of action should be to

A   call her back and ask her what is the matter
B   respect her wish not to talk about the incident
C   follow her into the bathroom
D   report in the nursing records that she has developed an incontinence problem

135   Which of the following should be the nursing action that day:

A   toilet her every 2 hours
B   restrict her fluids during the evening
C   observe for further episodes of incontinence
D   commence an intake and output chart

136   Which of the following instructions to night staff is most appropriate if Miss Thomas is incontinent again the following night:

A   offer her a commode by the bed
B   wake her 2 hourly during the night
C   nurse her on a Kylie absorbent incontinence sheet
D   do not give her a 10 pm drink

137   Later in the week Miss Thomas becomes constipated which adds to her distress. She has not had her bowels open for 3 days and is uncomfortable. She tells you that at home she is 'regular'. The nurse's first choice of action should be to

A   see that she is written up for a laxative
B   encourage her to take bran on her food
C   check that she is eating what she has at home
D   give her 2 glycerin suppositories

Mark your answers here: 134.......135.......136.......137.......

134 C 52%

This preserves her dignity yet allows her support if she is developing a new problem. A would only add to her embarassment, B is ignoring the situation and she will have received no reassurance and D is the wrong action without first assessing the situation.

135 C 84%

The first stage of the process is assessment. As this appears to be a new problem, complete assessment is needed before any planning can take place.

136 A 84%

As the most likely cause is her immobility in this new environment, A is the kindest and least humiliating choice if her bed cannot be moved any nearer to the toilets. If the problem persists then plans can be changed.

137 D 40%

As Miss Thomas is uncomfortable the priority is to ease her discomfort. Once that has been achieved a plan can be implemented which restores regularity.

Mobilising

Joseph Hickman is a forty year old publican; he is a balding, red faced obese gentleman. He is admitted to your surgical ward for stripping of his varicose veins. He also complains of chronic constipation.(RGN)

138 Joe is overheard chatting to another patient saying that he will be glad when the doctors have taken out the veins and he can have a good rest while his legs heal. What would the nurse deduce from this. That Joe

   A   is not unduly anxious and understands what is going to happen during his treatment
   B   has an obvious need for education regarding his condition
   C   is simply making social conversation with his neighbour
   D   is very anxious and is simply hiding his real feelings

139 Which of the following would be included in Joe's nursing care plan after his operation:

   A   restricted fluids, observation of wound sites, exercise, daily dressings
   B   high fluid intake, exercise, supportive bandages, observation of wound sites
   C   restricted fluids, rest, daily dressings, supportive bandages
   D   high fluid intake, rest, daily dressings, observation of wound site

140 If Joe was to adjust his life style to prevent a recurrence of his varicose veins then which of the following would need to be considered:

   A   alcohol, smoking, diet, medication
   B   smoking, diet, medication, elastic stockings
   C   alcohol, exercise, diet, elastic stockings
   D   smoking, exercise, diet, elastic stockings

Mark your answers here: 138.......139.......140.......

Answers

138 B 72%

Joe must be advised of the need to develop a collateral circulation after the operation so he can cooperate by walking the required distance each day.

139 B 90%

Restricted fluids would contribute to haemoconcentration and so increase the likelihood of clotting in the veins. Exercise and supportive bandages would help development of collateral circulation.

140 D 70%

Joe should be advised to avoid obesity and smoking, to wear elastic stockings and to exercise.

Mr James Blydon, a building contractor, has fallen from some scaffolding and sustained a left simple supracondylar fracture of the femoral shaft. He has had a Thomas splint applied in the Accident and Emergency Department and is to be treated conservatively.(RGN)

141 The sequence of events that occurs in the healing of fractures is

    A   remodelling, haematoma, callus formation, fibrous union
    B   fibrous union, callus formation, haematoma, remodelling
    C   callus formation, haematoma, fibrous union, remodelling
    D   haematoma, fibrous union, callus formation, remodelling

142 Skeletal traction is applied to Mr Blydon's leg via a Steinman's pin. Which of the following provides for the counter-traction:

    A   raising the foot of the bed with the aid of blocks
    B   attaching weights, through pulleys, to the ring of the Thomas splint
    C   attaching the splint to a Balkan beam
    D   raising the Thomas splint to 45 degrees

143 The method by which Mr Blydon will gain some of the lost strength in his limb in order to prepare for a walking caliper is with

    A   static quadriceps exercises
    B   dorsiflexion and plantarflexion of his foot
    C   flexion and extension of his knee
    D   increasing the traction weights

144 Mr Blydon is allowed to mobilise gently in a full length walking caliper. Which of the following best describes the function of the caliper. It will:

    A   keep the limb immobilised, yet allow movement
    B   allow him to walk without the fracture site taking any weight
    C   permit a limited amount of walking
    D   allow him to walk and test the fracture site for stability

Mark your answers here: 141.......142.......143.......144.......

141 D 93%

The first stage is haematoma where the bone ends eventually become 'sticky' and allow for fibrous union when threads temporarily form across the fracture and pave the way for callus formation. New bone is both replaced and fashioned by remodelling, a process which may take many months to complete.

142 A 57%

Although the ring of the Thomas splint is often attached, through pulleys to weights, this is done to allow the patient greater movement in bed. The counter-traction is provided by the patient's own weight pulling against the raised end of the bed. In effect, raising the splint would have a similar effect but 45 degrees would be too uncomfortable.

143 A 65%

The area of the greatest loss in power will be his thigh and because he cannot move this part static quadriceps exercises (i.e. strengthening exercises without movement of the joints) will be taught by the physiotherapist and encouraged by the nurses.

144 B 40%

The full length, (non weight-bearing) caliper is designed to transfer the weight from the foot, through metal rods, to the hip and thus by-pass the fracture site. Knee pads prevent the flexion of the knee and keep the limb straight, but not immobile.

4 : ELIMINATING

Susan aged 3 months is admitted to your ward with diarrhoea and vomiting. She is the first baby of teenage parents, has been fed on demand, is failing to thrive, and her genital area is excoriated.(RGN)

145 Which of the following is most important when caring for the intravenous infusion which the doctor erects, and asks to run at 20 ml per hour:

    A   maintain an intact dressing over the infusion site
    B   prevent accidental displacement of the needle
    C   observe the infusion site for signs of phlebitis
    D   ensure the infusion runs at the correct rate

146 Susan's condition steadily improves until 24 hours after admission you notice that her pulse rate is rising and she is becoming increasingly breathless. The appropriate course of action is to

    A   elevate her head and shoulders and take her temperature
    B   slow down the infusion rate and call the doctor
    C   suction her nasopharynx and administer oxygen
    D   check her blood pressure every 15 minutes

147 The correct daily fluid intake for Susan who weighs 4.5 kilograms is

    A   450 ml
    B   675 ml
    C   800 ml
    D   1000 ml

148 The best treatment for Susan's genital area, which is excoriated because of napkin dermatitis is to

    A   nurse her without nappies
    B   avoid the use of soap
    C   cleanse the area with soap and water and apply a steroid cream
    D   cleanse the area with oil and apply a barrier cream

Mark your answers here: 145.......146.......147.......148.......

145 D   76%

Although all other options are important, the one that can endanger Susan's life is D. If the infusion rate runs too quickly, she can very quickly get an overloaded circulation. Her total circulating volume is in the region of 450 ml.

146 B   73%

As Susan has been improving steadily until now, the chances are that the rise in pulse rate and increasing breathlessness, are due to overloading. Elevating her head and shoulders may help a little, but will not treat the cause. The doctor must be informed.

147 B   69%

Susan requires 150 ml per kilogram of weight.

148 A   61%

Once the skin is broken, barrier creams cannot be applied properly. Using steroids is contra-indicated as it can cause thinning of the skin. Most nappy rashes dry up and heal quickly if the air is allowed to get to the area, and if the area is no longer in contact with urine or faeces.

Sarah Gilbert is a **20** year old university student undertaking her first year examinations. She has recently experienced episodes of severe diarrhoea and has been admitted to a medical ward for treatment of ulcerative colitis. She is anxious and unwell.(RGN)

149 Sarah is most likely to have complained of

   A   pale stools, loss of weight, bleeding per rectum
   B   formed stools, blood and mucus in faeces, lassitude
   C   frequency of stools, weight loss, abdominal pain
   D   watery stools, anorexia, anal ulcers

150 Which of the following nursing actions should be taken when Sarah wishes to have her bowels open:

   A   give her a bedpan in bed
   B   tell her to use the nearby toilet
   C   provide a commode by her bed
   D   assist her to a commode in a private place

151 Which of the following nursing actions would be most useful in aiding Sarah's recovery:

   A   arrange diversional therapy to reduce her anxiety
   B   promote an environment for mental and physical rest
   C   place her near a toilet to reduce her embarrassment
   D   put her in a side room where she can study

152 The nurse should be prepared to explain the following investigations to Sarah:

   A   proctoscopy and faecal fat collection
   B   sigmoidoscopy and barium enema
   C   laparoscopy and barium meal
   D   colonoscopy and faecal stercobilinogen estimation

Mark your answers here: 149.......150.......151.......152.......

149 C   77%

All these are abnormal and are the main problems of a person with this disorder.

150 D   79%

This is the *most* satisfactory of the alternatives. As near to normality as possible and provides privacy and reduces stress. It is essential that the stool consistency and frequency is closely monitored.

151 B   64%

This is the most effective of the alternatives as a principle of care. The other alternatives are implicit in this answer.

152 B   89%

Both are undertaken for diagnostic purposes.

Mr William Hays, aged 68 years, has returned to the surgical ward from theatre after having had a transurethral resection of prostate gland. He has continuous bladder drainage in progress and catheter drainage is heavily blood stained.(RGN)

153 Which of the following groups of symptoms is Mr Hays most likely to have suffered from, before his operation:

A frequency, poor stream, dribbling
B polyuria, abdominal pain, dribbling
C dehydration, polyuria, thirst
D frequency, high blood urea, incontinence

154 Which of the following best describes the amount of fluid Mr Hays will be encouraged to drink after his continuous irrigation is discontinued, and the catheter drainage is no longer heavily blood stained:

A 3 litres per day, or more
B up to 500 ml per day as a maximum
C 15 ml hourly
D 500 ml hourly at least

155 Mrs Hays asks when Mr Hays is likely to be discharged home. The most appropriate answer is as soon as

A the catheter is removed
B good control of bladder is established
C the sutures are removed
D Mr Hays is fully mobile again

156 Mr Hays asks you if sexual performance will be affected by the operation. Which of the following would be the most appropriate answer:

A it is likely that he will lose the desire for sex, as the lack of hormones takes effect
B he will gradually become less able as the lack of hormones takes effect
C he should return to normal sexual activity at once
D he should return to normal sexual activity in about three weeks

Mark your answers here: 153.......154.......155.......156.......

153 A   92%

The symptoms can be understood in terms of the mechanisms of obstruction of the urinary outflow. Frequency occurs rather than polyuria, as the latter suggests large amounts of urine which is not the case. Abdominal pain occurs when the chronic obstruction becomes acute and no urine is passed at all. High blood urea is a sign not a symptom.

154 A   96%

It is important that Mr Hays' urinary output is kept high once the continuous irrigation is discontinued. Therefore a high level of oral fluids must be maintained. Three litres a day is regarded as a minimum for this purpose.

155 B   63%

Following removal of the catheter (at about 48 hours after the operation) bladder training is commenced to help Mr Hays gain full control. Mr Hays should be mobile soon after the operation to minimise the hazards of immobility, especially in a 68 year old. There are no sutures to remove following transurethral resection of prostate.

156 D   85%

Removal of the prostate gland should have no effect on sexual performance although Mr Hays will be unlikely to father children. However, following prostate surgery, strenuous exercise should be avoided for about three weeks.

Mr Fairfax is 65 years old and has suffered from chronic renal failure for some years. He has been admitted to hospital for terminal care.(RGN)

157 Mr Fairfax is likely to be anaemic because

    A   haematuria over many years has caused iron loss
    B   anorexia has caused insufficient iron intake
    C   red blood cell manufacture is reduced
    D   intestinal oedema causes poor absorption of iron

158 Which of the following is the reason why Mr Fairfax is likely to be uraemic:

    A   changes in the proximal tubule mean that urea is being re-absorbed
    B   glomerular filtration is impossible
    C   the number of functioning nephrons is reduced
    D   osmotic gradients between the tubule and efferent vessel cause urea reabsorption

159 A junior nurse asks you what Mr Fairfax's creatinine clearance test indicates. The test indicates

    A   the amount of blood filtered by the tubule, thus showing tubular reabsorption
    B   the efficiency of the distal convoluted tubule in controlling sodium and creatinine levels in the blood
    C   the amount of creatinine filtered throughout a 24 hour period, thus showing glomerular filtration rate
    D   the efficiency of the counter current mechanism around the loop of Henle

Mark your answers here: 157.......158.......159.......

157   C   72%

Red blood cell manufacture (erythropoiesis) is reduced due to lack of erythropoietin. This hormone is normally secreted by the kidneys but because of his renal failure Mr Fairfax has a deficiency of erythropoietin.

158   C   52%

The number of functioning nephrons is reduced in chronic renal failure. The remaining nephrons are able to filter, but they are insufficient in number to filter all the renal artery blood. Hence urea will remain unfiltered and recirculate causing uraemia.

159   C   74%

Creatinine is a waste product of cell metabolism and is completely filtered by the glomerulus. Only negligible amounts are reabsorbed by the tubule so that blood and urine creatinine levels are almost equal. If blood creatinine levels are higher than 24 hour urine levels then poor glomerular filtration is indicated.

Mrs Jones, a 33 year old wife and mother of three young children has been admitted to hospital for renal function tests, following several severe bouts of acute nephritis.(RGN)

160 **The reason why Mrs Jones will require bowel preparation for an intravenous pyelogram or urogram is**

    A   because a full rectum obscures the kidneys on X-ray
    B   because the patient may have her bowels open whilst being X-rayed
    C   to remove gas from the small intestine
    D   so that the kidneys are not obscured by faecal residue in the colon

161 **After being given frusemide Mrs Jones will need to micturate after**

    A   5-10 minutes
    B   20-30 minutes
    C   50-60 minutes
    D   an hour

162 **Investigations show that Mrs Jones has a renal stone for which a partial nephrectomy is done. Which of the following would normally be found in her urine postoperatively:**

    A   blood and glucose
    B   casts and stone fragments
    C   pus and stone fragments
    D   blood and protein

Mark your answers here: 160.......161.......162

160 D 64%

The right and left colonic flexures lie anterior to the kidneys, and if filled with radio-opaque substances such as gas or faeces, will obscure the kidneys and make the investigation worthless.

161 B 90%

Frusemide is a rapid acting potent loop diuretic (in 20-30 minutes).

162 D 82%

The cut area of the kidney is likely to bleed slightly, blood is protein and therefore protein and blood will be found postoperatively in her urine.

5 : COMMUNICATING

5 year old Nicky has left-sided otitis media, which did not respond to his family doctor's treatment. He is admitted to the children's ward for myringotomy, accompanied by his mother.(EN)

163 The condition of otitis media is

    A   an infection of the auditory meatus
    B   an inner ear infection
    C   a middle ear infection
    D   an infection of the mastoid bone

164 The correct position for Nicky to adopt whilst in bed in the first 24 hours after operation is

    A   on his left side
    B   supine
    C   on his right side
    D   prone

165 Which of the following items of advice would be appropriate to promoting Nicky's continued recovery when he goes home:

    A   keep his ears clean
    B   do not allow water to get into his ears
    C   discourage his participation in games at school
    D   promote oral hygiene

Mark your answers here: 163.......164.......165.......

163 C 88%

Otitis media is a middle ear infection. This is frequently carried from the tonsils via the pharyngeal (Eustachian) tube. In children the chronic disorder is often referred to as 'glue ear'.

164 A 54%

The operation of myringotomy (making an incision into the tympanic membrane) is performed to drain the middle ear cavity of infected fluid. Therefore positioning Nicky on his left side will promote drainage.

165 B 68%

Water entering his ear may carry infection with it into the middle ear.

Mr Alan Jones is in hospital to have surgical treatment for cataracts which affect both his eyes. He is aged seventy-five years and has had deteriorating sight for the last three years. Mr Jones appears to be depressed; he has been living alone since his wife died six months ago but is immaculately dressed and has brought a neatly packed suitcase containing essential personal items.(EN)

166   An accurate description of the condition affecting Mr Jones' eyes is that

   A   the retina has deteriorated with age
   B   the pressure in the eye is too high
   C   the lens of the eye has become opaque
   D   there has been a haemorrhage in the eye

167   Which of the following is the correct explanation to give Mr Jones about why he will need spectacles after the operation? These spectacles will

   A   magnify the image seen
   B   focus the image on the retina
   C   reduce the light rays entering the eye
   D   increase the light rays entering the eye

168   With reference to Mr Jones' antibiotic eye drops it is important that

   A   the same bottle is used for both eyes
   B   the drops are stored at room temperature
   C   a separate bottle is used for each eye
   D   the eye drops are instilled at the outer canthus

   Mark your answers here: 166.......167.......168.......

166 C 84%

Cataract is an opacity of the lens. A is retinopathy, B is glaucoma, D is hyphaemia.

167 B 41%

The lens is the part of the eye that has been removed. The function of the lens is to focus the image on the retina, replacement spectacles therefore perform this function. A, there is no point in a large unfocused image. C and D the pupil controls light entering the eye.

168 C 76%

Separate bottles are used to prevent transmission of infection. A is unsafe, it can transmit infection. Antibiotic drugs should be stored in a refrigerator, eye drops instilled at the outer canthus will trickle out of the eye.

Mrs Evelyn Groves, who is aged 71 years and lives alone, is attending the eye clinic because of chronic glaucoma. She is having problems coping at home because of her deteriorating vision.(EN)

169 When Mrs Groves asks you why her vision is deteriorating your best explanation to her is

    A   "the lens of your eye is clouding over"
    B   "the retina of your eye is slowly wearing out"
    C   "the pressure in your eye is higher than normal"
    D   "the pressure in your eye is lower than normal"

170 Which of the following treatments is likely to help control the chronic glaucoma:

    A   antibiotic drops
    B   removal of the lens
    C   drops that dilate the pupil
    D   drops that constrict the pupil

171 Which of the following people can best assess Mrs Groves' need for aids to help her at home, and arrange for these aids to be supplied:

    A   the home help
    B   the health visitor
    C   the occupational therapist
    D   the ophthalmic technician

172 If Mrs Groves is prescribed eye drops and she cannot instil them herself, then the most appropriate person to help her with this task is

    A   the health visitor
    B   the general practitioner
    C   community nurse
    D   social worker

Mark your answers here: 169.......170.......171.......172.......

169 C 69%

Glaucoma is raised intra-ocular pressure. A is a cataract, B, retinopathy, D is likely to occur due to dehydration.

170 D 44%

Drops that constrict the pupil help glaucoma because they improve drainage of the aqueous humour from the eye. A, are for infection, B is only helpful for cataract and C, dilating the pupil reduces the aqueous drainage from the eye and so is counter-productive.

171 C 80%

This is the role of the occupational therapist. The home help can help in practical ways but does not have the special training needed to assess needs in this area. The health visitor is concerned with maintenance of health and does not have the appropriate skills to assess need for aids. The ophthalmic technician prepares equipment for ophthalmologists and ophthalmic surgeons.

172 C 88%

The community nurse is the only member of the primary health care team whose role is to offer practical nursing help.

John Medlan has been going deaf for a number of months and has been admitted for stapedectomy.(RGN)

173 **The type of deafness from which John is suffering is**

    A   conductive
    B   nerve
    C   perceptive
    D   vestibular

174 **Which of the following is the period of time when John can expect his hearing to return after the operation:**

    A   after one or two weeks
    B   immediately
    C   after one month
    D   in about three months

175 **Which of the following may be used to replace the stapes:**

    A   donor stapes
    B   a steel wire piston
    C   a bone graft
    D   a plug of fat

176 **Which of the following will be included in John's postoperative care:**

    A   irrigate the ear
    B   dry mop the ear
    C   prevent coughing
    D   instil antibiotic ear drops

Mark your answers here: 173.......174.......175.......176.......

173 A   82%

The stapes is one of the auditory ossicles which conduct sound across the middle ear. There is no nerve involvement, and John has no problems with perception.

174 B   53%

Stapedectomy is usually performed for otosclerosis and the operation provides immediate restoration of ossicular movement which provides immediate return of hearing.

175 B   46%

A piece of wire is used to connect the incus with the oval window.

176 C   57%

Coughing produces pressure changes within the middle ear which can cause movement of the prosthesis.

Mrs Mills, aged 40 years, is recovering from a pulmonary embolism, a complication that she developed following surgery. She is to continue with anticoagulant therapy, i.e. warfarin, after her discharge from hospital.(EN)

177 Which of the following is the antidote to warfarin:

    A   vitamin K
    B   protamine sulphate
    C   vitamin E
    D   protamine zinc

178 Which of the following groups of medications should Mrs Mills be advised to avoid whilst taking warfarin:

    A   alcohol, Dorbanex, paracetamol
    B   Dorbanex, paracetamol, contraceptive pill
    C   contraceptive pill, aspirin, alcohol
    D   aspirin, alcohol, Dorbanex

179 Which of the following observations will Mrs Mills be advised to make in order to detect problems after discharge. To look for

    A   urinary infection, headaches
    B   headaches, bruising
    C   bruising, excessive bleeding
    D   excessive bleeding, urinary infection

180 Which of the following are most likely to be responsible for Mrs Mills' warfarin control after her discharge home:

    A   pathology department and general practitioner
    B   health centre only
    C   health centre and out-patient department
    D   pathology department only

Mark your answers here: 177.......178.......179.......180.......

Answers

177 A 57%

Vitamin K is the specific antidote to warfarin, while protamine sulphate is the specific antidote to heparin.

178 C 61%

The contraceptive pill can increase the susceptibility to clot formation, and aspirin and alcohol enhance the action of warfarin.

179 C 69%

A tendency to bleeding would require the dosage of anticoagulants to be adjusted.

180 A 61%

The pathology department will prescribe the required dosage of warfarin and the general practitioner will provide the prescription for the tablets.

Mr Ian Matthews, a **28** year old widower, is admitted to the ward via the Accident and Emergency Department, at **16.00** hours, following a road traffic accident on his way to collect his two children aged **6** and **7** years from school. He has suspected abdominal injuries and is to go to theatre at **17.00** hours for exploratory surgery under general anaesthesia. He has an intravenous infusion of dextrose/saline in progress which is maintaining a normal circulating fluid volume.(EN)

181 Which of the following would be of most concern to Mr Matthews prior to theatre. The:

    A   care of his children
    B   severity of his condition
    C   time he will be in hospital
    D   long-term effects of his injuries

182 The most appropriate initial nursing action to take when Mr Matthews' infusion ceases to flow is to

    A   open the flow rate control until flow is re-started
    B   re-position his arm
    C   inform the doctor
    D   flush the intravenous cannula with heparin

183 On routine urinalysis you would expect to find

    A   straw coloured, specific gravity 1010, pH 6.5
    B   protein, specific gravity 1015, pH 9
    C   albumin, straw coloured, specific gravity 1005
    D   pH 4, acetone, specific gravity 1010

184 Which of the following would concern you most when you recorded Mr Matthews' half hourly routine observations:

    A   increasing pain, rising blood pressure
    B   falling pulse, rising blood pressure
    C   falling urinary output, increasing pain
    D   falling blood pressure, rising pulse

Mark your answers here: 181.......182.......183.......184.......

Answers

181 A   66%

B, C and D are all connected with A. The main concern a young father would have in this situation would be the welfare of his children, both immediate and long-term.

182 B   58%

This is the first and basic course of action. Most often the infusion will not run because the flow is obstructed by the cannula being in position to occlude the end of the vein, or the vein being in spasm, by contra-gravitational forces or by the limb being cold causing vasoconstriction. Most of the common causes are resolved by re-positioning the limb.

183 A   86%

This is a normal urinalysis. As there is no indication of definite trauma one would not expect to find any abnormal results. The circulating volume has been maintained by intravenous infusion and so a high specific gravity is not expected. Trauma to the kidney has not been identified so filtration is expected to be normal, there will be no albumin or protein in the urine.

184 D   64%

The probable reason for this is that Mr Matthews is becoming shocked, probably because of internal bleeding. This is a life-threatening situation.

Following a gas explosion, Mr Kevin Thorton is admitted having received severe burns to his chest and both arms. Mr Thornton is 40 years old, married with two teenage children.(RGN)

185 Which of the following best represents the likely amount of skin surface area involved in Mr Thornton's burns:

    A   25% of body surface
    B   36% of body surface
    C   48% of body surface
    D   55% of body surface

186 The probable reason why Mr Thornton may require eye drops during the first few days is in order to

    A   treat the conjunctivitis caused by the flash
    B   keep the pupils dilated for examination
    C   clear the dust caused by the explosion
    D   provide 'false tears' needed because of dehydration

187 Which of the following would Mr Thornton need if his burns are to be treated using the 'open' method:

    A   sterile bedsheets, barrier nursing, no dressings
    B   open all dressings, apply fan therapy, prick blisters
    C   cover area with sterile dressings that are opened daily for short periods
    D   wounds are opened surgically to allow new growth of skin

188 Mr Thornton asks about the pain he will have following skin grafting. The most accurate reply would be that

    A   analgesia will control his pain totally
    B   the burned area will be painful, but analgesia will help
    C   the donor area will be painful but analgesia will help
    D   skin grafts are usually pain-free

Mark your answers here: 185.......186.......187.......188.......

185 B   78%

Wallace's 'rules of nine' provide a good estimate of surface area involved. In adults the following percentages apply: head 9%, front of torso 18%, back of torso 18%, arms 9% each, legs 18% each (upper leg 9% lower 9%), genital area 1%. Therefore in Mr Thornton's case he has his front 18%, plus 2 arms (each 9%) 18%, giving 36% in all.

186 D   62%

Due to the severe fluid loss, the lacrimal apparatus may not produce sufficient fluid to keep the conjuctiva moist. Scarring of the conjunctiva can ensue if adequate moisture is not provided by regular instillation of 'artificial tears'.

187 A   88%

The 'open method' involves allowing the wounds to form 'crusts' and 'eschar' (dead tissue) within 48-72 hours. Eschar may need to be removed surgically as infection can occur beneath it. Partial thickness burns may well heal under crusts but full-thickness burns usually require skin grafts ultimately.

188 C   76%

It would be false to promise Mr Thornton a completely pain-free postoperative period. The donor site is often the most painful for patients because raw nerve endings are exposed when the split graft is taken.

Edna Hill is a 69 year old widow who lives alone. She is a keen gardener and enjoys outings with her children and grandchildren. She has been suffering from stress incontinence for some time and has recently been diagnosed as having a cystocele. Edna is admitted to hospital for an anterior colporrhaphy. (RGN)

189 Which of the following causes the decreased elasticity of vaginal tissue in postmenopausal women, which predisposes to vaginal prolapse:

    A   less progesterone in circulation
    B   less oestrogen in circulation
    C   more oestrogen in circulation
    D   more progesterone in circulation

190 Which of the following is most important when planning Edna's care in the first 48 hours after operation? Edna:

    A   may have a urethral catheter *in situ*
    B   is likely to be sick
    C   needs a low fibre diet
    D   may become confused after the anaesthetic

191 Postoperatively Edna is most likely to develop

    A   urinary infection
    B   pulmonary embolism
    C   paralytic ileus
    D   chest infection

192 The most important piece of advice to give Edna before she goes home is

    A   to rest in bed each afternoon
    B   not to lift heavy weights for several weeks
    C   to visit her doctor as soon as possible
    D   not to take a high fibre diet

Mark your answers here: 189.......190.......191.......192.......

189 B 77%

B is the only correct answer.

190 A 76%

Edna may or may not have a urethral catheter but if she has not then a special watch needs to be kept on her urinary output.

191 A 70%

The bladder is in close proximity to the area of operation, and bruising may cause Edna to have some residual urine in her bladder following micturition. This gives ideal conditions for a urinary infection to develop.

192 B 96%

If Edna lifts heavy weights before her pelvic floor has healed she may develop a uterine prolapse which may cause major problems and result in a second operation.

Mrs Jane Evans, aged 41 years, is admitted to the ward for a total abdominal hysterectomy for prolonged menorrhagia. She lives with her husband and has two children aged thirteen and ten.(RGN)

193   Which of the following are removed when a total abdominal hysterectomy is performed? The

    A   body of uterus
    B   uterus and cervix
    C   uterus and ovaries
    D   uterus and uterine tubes

194   The most important investigation for Mrs Evans to have is a

    A   haemoglobin count
    B   high vaginal swab
    C   mid-stream specimen of urine
    D   pelvic examination

195   The most likely complication after Mrs Evans' operation is

    A   haemorrhage
    B   urinary retention
    C   infection
    D   severe depression

196   Which of the following is the nurse most likely to be asked to collect when Mrs Evans develops a pyrexia following the operation:

    A   sputum specimen and wound swab
    B   wound swab and high vaginal swab
    C   mid-stream specimen of urine and wound swab
    D   sputum specimen and mid-stream specimen of urine

Mark your answers here: 193.......194.......195.......196.......

193 B   62%

Before the risks of carcinoma of the cervix were documented the cervix was left *in situ* and only the body of the uterus removed. Now both are usually removed.

194 A   82%

A low haemoglobin is likely in a patient with menorrhagia and is potentially hazardous in a patient undergoing surgery. The other investigations may be carried out but are not the most important.

195 B   69%

Urinary retention is the most likely complication as the bladder and urethra are often bruised during the operation.

196 C   83%

Urine infections are common complications of hysterectomy and wound infections may also occur. Although a high vaginal swab may be taken this is not the most likely.

Margaret Carpenter aged 42 is married with two grown up daughters. Recently she started to have very heavy menstrual periods for which the cause has been diagnosed as fibroids. Her doctor suggests that she should have a hysterectomy.(RGN)

197 Which of the following will be true about Margaret after her operation? She will:

    A   have the same level of libido
    B   be less interested in sex
    C   have hot flushes
    D   gain weight

198 Which of the following will increase the risk of Margaret suffering from a deep venous thrombosis following her operation:

    A   discontinuing hormone preparations
    B   smoking
    C   varicose veins
    D   sensible dieting pre-operatively

199 The most appropriate piece of advice to give to Margaret before her discharge is that

    A   she should avoid fibre in the diet for three months
    B   she should avoid exercise for three months
    C   she should take increasing amounts of exercise for three months
    D   she may expect vaginal loss for three months

Mark your answers here: 197.......198.......199.......

197 A   51%

A is the right answer and can be confirmed by research findings. C is only the case if the ovaries are removed. D is only correct if the patient takes little exercise and over-eats after the hysterectomy.

198 C   40%

C is the right answer because of the delayed venous return caused by congestion. A would be more of a concern if the patient continued to take certain hormone preparations. B is more likely to put the patient at risk of a chest infection. D is not a hazard unless the patient has been crash dieting in which case her general health may have suffered.

199 C   48%

C is the correct answer as Margaret will be very tired when she leaves the hospital but needs to get back to normal. A is only correct if Margaret has some disorder of the bowel. D is incorrect, patients have a vaginal loss for about two weeks after the operation, but if it were to continue for three months it might indicate failure of healing.

Mrs Joan Ellis, a 40 year old housewife with two teenage children, is going to have a hysterectomy in two days time. She was diagnosed as having a submucus uterine fibroid two months ago.(RGN)

200 Which of the following would be most likely to give rise to some of Mrs Ellis' symptoms:

    A   pressure on other pelvic organs
    B   anaemia from recurrent bleeding
    C   chronic infection of urine
    D   psychological problems of the menopause

201 In the first few days after the operation Mrs Ellis has difficulty in passing urine. Which would be the most appropriate nursing action:

    A   to encourage Mrs Ellis to drink extra fluids, and explain that it may take a few days for her bladder to return to normal
    B   to tell Mrs Ellis that she will soon be well, but she must not worry about the problem
    C   to advise Mrs Ellis to forget about it, and only visit the toilet when she feels desperate
    D   to persuade Mrs Ellis to socialise with other patients, so that they may discuss common problems

202 On the tenth day following her operation, Mrs Ellis complains of substernal pain and shortage of breath. The most likely cause of this problem is

    A   chest infection
    B   heartburn
    C   indigestion
    D   pulmonary embolism

Mark your answers here: 200.......201.......202.......

200 B 70%

Mrs Ellis' main complaint will probably be tiredness and lethargy, caused by anaemia. A submucus fibroid is situated under the endometrium, so it would be unlikely to give rise to pressure symptoms unless it was exceptionally large.

201 A 93%

Extra fluids will minimise the possibility of urinary infection whilst Mrs Ellis has some residual urine in her bladder. Disturbance of the area of the operation is the cause of the problem and will eventually settle down.

202 D 80%

Deep venous thrombosis and pulmonary embolism are classical complications of gynaecological operations because of the interference with the venous drainage of her legs during the operation.

Carol and David are a young couple about to get married. They discuss methods of contraception together, and with their general practitioner. It is decided that Carol should take Eugynon, a combined contraceptive pill. (RGN)

203 The correct regime for Carol to follow when taking the pill is

    A   every day, irrespective of menstruation
    B   21 days, then 7 days without the pill
    C   28 days, then 7 days without the pill
    D   every day, until she menstruates

204 Which of the following is the correct information to give Carol about how the pill acts:

    A   it inhibits ovulation
    B   it prevents fertilisation
    C   sperm are prevented from reaching the ovum
    D   fertilised ovum cannot implant in the uterus

205 One month after starting to take the pill, Carol visits the clinic complaining of early morning sickness. The couple have been using a condom each time they have intercourse. The most appropriate advice to give to Carol is

    A   that if she does not have a period soon, she is likely to be pregnant
    B   not to worry, it could be a 'tummy upset', or something she has eaten
    C   that the nausea is a side-effect of the pill, and will probably settle down
    D   the couple should think about using a different contraception

206 Which of the following would cause the greatest concern:

    A   the couple had a night out and Carol took the pill 4 hours later than usual
    B   Carol's period was two days late and it only lasted for one day
    C   at a routine clinic visit, Carol has gained 8 lb in weight and her blood pressure is 146/90 mm Hg
    D   Carol notices a slight, white discharge

Mark your answers here: 203.......204.......205.......206.......

203 B 92%

The 7 days when Carol omits to take the pill allow her hormone levels to fall low enough to allow her to 'menstruate'. She takes the pill for 21 days, and allows 7 days for menstruation, thus mimicking a normal 28 day cycle.

204 A 78%

The combined contraceptive pill inhibits ovulation by maintaining high levels of female hormones. Progesterone-only pills inhibit fertilisation, as do barrier methods of contraception. The intrauterine device prevents implantation of the fertilised ovum.

205 C 79%

The doctor may perform a pregnancy test as a precaution, but since the couple have been using another method of contraception, the possibility of pregnancy is small. At this stage reassurance is appropriate since nausea may occur, but usually settles down.

206 C 86%

Weight gain can be a major problem with oral contraception, and hypertension, linked with the increased possibility of deep vein thrombosis would give rise for concern. Answer A would be a problem with the progesterone-only pill, and B and D may not be normal.

Mrs Anne Jones, aged 22 years, is admitted to your ward during the night, in a collapsed state with a ruptured ectopic pregnancy. She is accompanied by her husband.(RGN)

207 The most likely cause of collapse in an ectopic pregnancy is

A hypovolaemic shock
B cardiogenic shock
C anaphylaxis
D septicaemia

208 Which of the following is the most common time in the pregnancy for an ectopic pregnancy to rupture:

A before the fourth week of pregnancy
B between the sixth and twelfth week
C between the sixteenth and twentieth week
D between the twelfth and sixteenth week

209 Which of the following would the nurse expect Mrs Jones to undergo prior to an emergency operation:

A abdominal shave, enema, blood transfusion
B abdominal shave, pelvic examination, intravenous infusion
C pubic shave, enema, blood transfusion
D pubic shave, pelvic examination, intravenous infusion

210 Which of the following is most appropriate for Mr Jones, before his wife goes to theatre. He should be

A given the ward name, telephone number and sent home
B allowed to stay in the waiting room
C given the ward telephone number and sent for toilet articles
D allowed to stay at his wife's bedside

Mark your answers here: 207.......208.......209.......210.......

207 A 85%

The patient haemorrhages into the pelvic cavity because of the rupture of blood vessels in the wall of the ovarian tube, as the embryo enlarges. The wall has a particularly rich blood supply during the early stages of pregnancy.

208 B 86%

It is impossible for a pregnancy to continue in the uterine tube much beyond the tenth week of gestation because of the limited capacity for expansion in the tube.

209 B 35%

Abdominal shave would be performed as Mrs Jones would have a laparotomy. A pelvic examination would be performed by the doctor to exclude any other condition, and an intravenous infusion is essential prior to a blood transfusion. A plasma expander such as Haemaccel may be used.

210 D 74%

Mr and Mrs Jones are both likely to be very distressed, and the husband will be concerned for his wife's welfare. By being together they can support each other during this crisis.

Miss Flyde is 77 years old. She is admitted to your ward for terminal care with a fungating cancer of the breast with widespread metastases. Until her admission she was looked after by her only relative, a 70 year old sister, with support from the district nurse. On admission Miss Flyde is ambulant, but in considerable pain and suffering from cachexia.(RGN)

211   Which of the following definitions would you use if you were explaining the meaning of the word cachexia to a junior nurse:

A   bad breath
B   loss of appetite
C   malnutrition and wasting
D   loss of hair on the head

212   Miss Flyde's pain is being controlled by an oral preparation of strong analgesics, which is given four hourly, and generally seems to be effective. When you go to administer the medicine at 10 am, Miss Flyde complains of feeling drowsy and nauseated. Which of the following courses of action would you take:

A   not give the medicine and telephone the doctor for instructions
B   give the medicine and reassure Miss Flyde that these symptoms are not significant
C   not give the medicine and inform the doctor when he visits the ward later
D   give the medicine and ask Miss Flyde to inform you if she does not improve

213   The probable reason for Miss Flyde's sister becoming increasingly demanding and generally difficult when she visits the ward is because

A   she feels that the nurses do not anticipate her sister's needs
B   she wants to care for her sister herself
C   she thinks her sister is not receiving adequate care
D   she cannot accept the consequences of her sister's illness

Mark your answers here: 211.......212.......213.......

211 C   91%

Cachexia is often caused by cancer. Halitosis means bad breath, anorexia is loss of appetite and alopecia means hair loss.

212 A   84%

If Miss Flyde is nauseated then the medication should not be given because it may increase the nausea and possibly cause vomiting. The doctor needs to be informed immediately so he can prescribe an alternative before Miss Flyde begins to experience pain.

213 D   75%

Miss Flyde's sister has to come to terms with the deterioration in the patient's condition, and the prospect of her death. This means that the surviving sister will be alone in the world, and she is looking for help and support at a very difficult time.